D0045701

LOW BACK
PAIN SYNDROME

by

RENE CAILLIET, M. D.

Chairman and Professor
Department of Rehabilitative Medicine
University of Southern California School of Medicine
Los Angeles, California

SECOND EDITION

 F. A. DAVIS *Company*

PHILADELPHIA

Also by Rene Cailliet:

SHOULDER PAIN

NECK AND ARM PAIN

FOOT AND ANKLE PAIN

HAND: PAIN AND IMPAIRMENT

KNEE PAIN AND DISABILITY

Copyright © 1968 by F. A. Davis Company

Second printing 1971
Third printing 1972
Fourth printing 1974
Fifth printing 1974
Sixth printing 1975
Seventh printing 1976
Eighth printing 1976
Ninth printing 1977
Tenth printing 1978

Printed in the United States of America

Preface

The low back pain syndrome affects probably 80 per cent of the members of the human race at some time in their lives. Although it rarely results in mortality, its morbidity is high, inconvenience great, and economic burden significant. In the past year, even the office of the President of the United States was disturbed by its presence! Its prevention is aided by posture training in the schools, safety engineering, and physical fitness consciousness in general.

In spite of awareness of the problem the feeling of inadequacy in evaluation and management of the complaint of "backache, low down" has been expressed by many competent physicians. The need for a simple practical text on low back pain has been voiced often by medical students, interns, and residents. It is in an effort to meet this apparent need that this book has been written and is offered as a working basis for the diagnosis and treatment of painful conditions of the low back. With a chapter on the functional anatomy and mechanical evaluation of the normal spine as a basis, an attempt has been made to point the way to evaluation of the spine in the patient having low back pain. Since the symptoms are due to mechanical malfunction in the vast majority of such patients, they lend themselves to evaluation and treatment if the normal mechanisms are known and deviations from the normal are recognized.

Because the *stick-man* type of illustration has proved valuable in blackboard talks to students in the class room, to physicians at staff meetings, and to the patient in the office it has been employed here to provide a simple and positive approach to a subject considered complex and controversial. It is hoped that these drawings together with the text will provide a blueprint for the diagnostician and therapist concerned with the patient complaining of low back pain. It is also hoped that the book will serve as an aid to the medical student in understanding the functional anatomy of the spine in both normal and abnormal conditions.

I am indebted to Dr. Sidney Licht for his encouragement and constructive criticism of the work, to the reviewers obtained by my publishers, and to my wife for typing and editing the manuscript as well as for her patience during the hours devoted to its composition.

RENE CAILLIET, M.D.

Table of Contents

Illustrations

CHAPTER 1

Anatomy

The complaint of pain in the low back is probably voiced at some period of life by 80 per cent of the members of the human race; in fact it is responsible for a large percentage of patients' visits to physicians. Fortunately, the vast majority of low back discomforts are of a "mechanical" origin. When properly evaluated they will respond to treatment directed toward correction of the mechanical impairment.

In the patient complaining of low back pain the interpretation of symptoms and the evaluation of the physical findings are surprisingly simplified when the examiner has a fundamental knowledge of functional anatomy. Appreciation of *functional* anatomy of the human spine in its normal state and evaluation of its deviation from normal in the symptomatic state are all important for successful treatment.

Any discussion referring to *mechanical* low back dysfunction or discomfort must eliminate the low back pain resulting from fracture, metastatic disease, metabolic disease, or diseases of viscera with symptoms referred to the region of the spine. Proper history taking, careful examination, and appropriate laboratory studies will usually reveal these non-mechanical conditions if their possibility is kept in mind.

FUNCTIONAL UNIT

The vertebral column, the supporting structure of erect two-legged man, affords *static* support and *kinetic* function. The human spine of the present-day man must be considered to be still in the evolutionary phase of adaptation of man's body to the forces of gravity.

It has not as yet adequately adapted to the ever-changing stresses to which man is being subjected and to which he is subjecting himself. However, man's spine, with its admitted anatomic and functional inadequacies, must be understood, evaluated, and aided in order to cope with the stresses imposed upon it by everyday activities. Functional adaptation of tomorrow's spine will not ease the burden of today's discomfort.

The evolution of man's posture is an incomplete study, and the anthropology of posture is a meager science. A study of the past will undoubtedly explain much of the posture of today, both in its adequacies and inadequacies. It is a fair assumption that our present-day concepts of posture could well be altered by studies of social customs, nationality differentiations, and cultural differences that have led to biologic adaptations. The anthropology of posture is a fertile field as yet uncultivated. A study of body mechanics may well elucidate the shortcomings of our ancestral heritage and its postural concepts and lead to a more comfortable and more functional use of man's spine based on sound principals rather than on folklore, faulty habit, and erroneous teaching.

The human spine is an aggregate of superimposed segments, each segment being a self-contained *functional unit*, with the sum total of all the units forming the vertebral column. The function of the spine is the support of a two-legged animal, man, in an upright position, defying gravity, conserving energy, and permitting locomotion and purposeful movement. Antigravity support and flexibility are two engineering feats that are demanded of the human spine.

The lumbar spine is a jointed column of superimposed hydraulic units, itself eccentrically loaded, yet capable of supporting large weights and dependent on the integrity of each unit for the integrity of its whole structure. Each functional unit must be structurally and functionally delineated before the large composite superstructure of the total spinal column is studied.

The functional unit is composed of two segments—the anterior segment containing two vertebral bodies, one superincumbent on the other, separated by a "disk," and the posterior segment consisting functionally of two articulations. The anterior segment is exclusively a supporting, weight-bearing, shock-absorbing structure, whereas the posterior segment is a non-weight-bearing structure the prime function of which is directional guidance (Fig. 1).

Anterior Portion of Functional Unit

The anterior portion of the functional unit is well constructed for its weight-bearing shock-absorbing function. The unit is comprised of two cylindrical vertebral bodies with flattened cephalic and caudal ends that, in their normal state, are adequate to sustain extremes of compressive stresses. These two vertebral bodies are separated by a hydraulic system called a disk.

At birth, the vertebral bodies are bi-convex with the end plates being cartilaginous. These cartilage plates gradually undergo ossification and from the age of 16 to 20 years fuse with the bony vertebra. This end plate is the point of attachment of the fibers of the annulus fibrosus and after puberty when ossification is completed the central and posterior aspect of the plate remain cartilaginous.

The disk is a self-contained fluid system that absorbs shock, permits transient compression, and, owing to fluid displacement within an elastic container, allows movement. It is quite evident then that the disk is a mechanical "shock absorber."

The anatomy of the disk lends itself well to its intended function. The upper and the lower plates of the disk are the end plates of the vertebral bodies. These plates are articular hyaline cartilage in direct contact and adherent to the underlying resilient bone of the vertebral body. In their normal state these end plates are firm, flat, circular, inflexible surfaces that form the cephalad and caudal portions of the disk and to which is attached the encircling annulus fibrosus.

The annulus, or wall, of the disk is an intertwining fibroelastic mesh that encapsulates the matrix of the disk. The matrix, or nucleus pulposus, is thus confined within a fibrous resilient wall, the annulus, and between a floor and

2

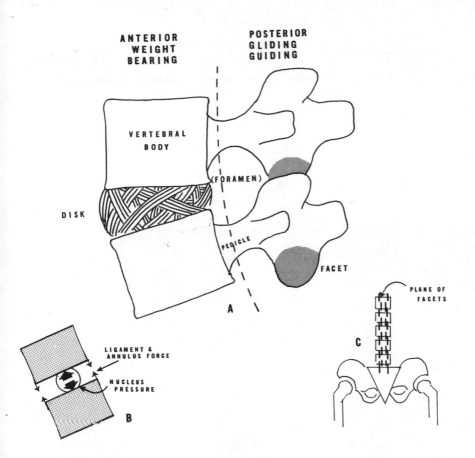

FIGURE 1. The *functional unit* of the spine in cross section. A, Lateral view. B depicts pressure within disk forcing vertebra apart and the balancing force of the long ligaments. C depicts the plane of the facets gliding motion.

ceiling composed of the end plates of the vertebrae. The annulus fibrils are attached around the entire circumference of both the upper and inferior vertebral bodies and crisscross and intertwine in oblique directions. The manner in which these semi-elastic fibers interwine permits movement of one vertebra upon the other in a rocker-like movement and to a lesser degree permits movement in a shearing direction (Fig. 2).

The fluid contained within the confines of the encircling annulus is a colloidal gel and by its self-contained fluidity has all the characteristics of a hydraulic system. Because the nucleus is approximately 80 per cent fluid,

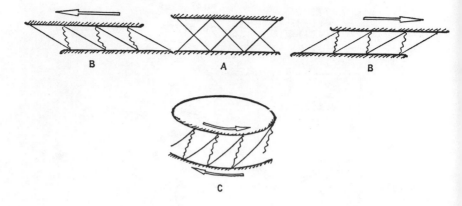

FIGURE 2. Elasticity of annulus fibers. A depicts the resting *functional unit* with all fibers taut. Lateral shear tightens half of the fibers and thus retains intradiskal tension (B). Similiar effect is noted on rotation in C.

it cannot itself be compressed but since it exists in a closed container it conforms to the law of Pascal, which states that: "Any external force exerted on a unit area of a confined liquid is transmitted undiminished to every unit area of the interior of the containing vessel" (Blaise Pascal, 1623-1662).

The self-contained fluid accepts the shock of a compression force attempting to approximate the two vertebrae and maintains the separation of the two vertebral bodies. Movement of one vertebra on the other in a rocking-like manner is permitted by the ability of the fluid to shift anteriorly or posteriorly within a semi-elastic container. The constant internal disk pressure separates the two end plates and thus keeps the fibro-elastic mesh of the annulus taut (Fig. 3).

The elastic properties of the disk are considered to reside in the elasticity of the annulus rather than in the fluid content of the nucleus. In a "young" and undamaged disk the fibroelastic tissue of the annulus is predominantly elastic. In the process of aging or as a residual of injury, there is a relative increase in the percentage of fibrous elements. As the relative increase of fibrous elements occurs, the disk loses its elasticity, and its recoil hydraulic mechanism decreases. The "older" annulus reveals a replacement of the highly elastic collagen fibrils by large fibrotic bands of collagen tissue devoid of mucoid material. This disk is, therefore, less elastic.

The nucleus pulposus is a colloidal gel, a muco-polysaccharide that has a physical-chemical action. In a "young" and in an undamaged disk the nucleus is 80 per cent water. Due to its colloidal chemical nature it can imbibe external fluids and maintain its intrinsic fluid balance. As the nucleus ages it loses its water-binding capacity. After the first two decades the nucleus water content decreases from its early 80 per cent because its water-binding capacity has been

4

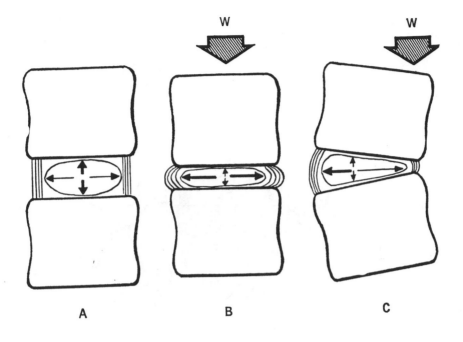

FIGURE 3. Hydraulic mechanism of the intervertebral disk. A, The normal resting disk with the internal pressure indicated by the arrows exerted in all directions. The disk is confined above and below by the vertebral plates and circumferentially by the annulus. The annulus fibers are taut. B, Compression of the disk is permitted by the non-compressible fluid of the nucleus expanding the annulus. Flexibility is seen to exist in the annulus. C, Flexion of the spine is permitted by horizontal shift of the nuclear fluid which maintains its cubic content but causes expansion of the posterior annulus and contraction of the anterior annulus. The intertwining of the annular fibers permits this change in the capsule with no loss of turgor.

decreased. In the aging process there is a decrease in the protein polysaccharide with an additional loss of osmotic and imbibition properties.

The intervertebral disk has a vascular supply that disappears after the second decade. By the third decade the disk, now avascular, receives its nutrition by diffusion of lymph through the vertebral end plates and by virtue of the physical-chemical imbibitory characteristics of the nucleus colloidal gel. The ability of an injured disk to regain its elasticity is bound to be stronger in the young.

Resistance to stress by the vertebral column is further augmented by the vertebral ligaments. The ligaments run longitudinally along the vertebral column and by their attachments restrict excessive movement of the unit in any direction and prevent any significant shearing action. The ligaments by their

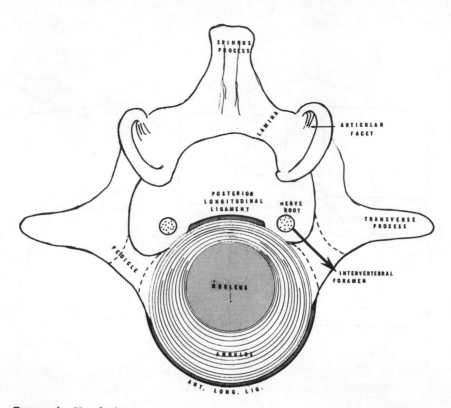

FIGURE 4. Vertebral segment. As viewed from above the vertebral segment is divided into the anterior and posterior segments. The anterior portion is the vertebral body and the disk structures. The posterior portion consists of the lamina, pedicles, facets, etc. In this segment the posterior longitudinal ligament is incomplete placing it at the lower lumbar (L_5) level.

position and attachments encase the disk and reinforce the annulus yet do not detract from its physiologic elasticity. Viewed at the level of the functional unit the entire disk is enclosed anteriorly by the anterior longitudinal ligament and posteriorly by the posterior longitudinal ligament; the disk encasement is completed posterolaterally by the pedicles of the vertebral arch (Fig. 4).

Of functional and potential pathologic significance is the fact that the posterior longitudinal ligament is intact throughout the entire length of the vertebral column until in its caudal approach it reaches the lumbar region. At the first lumbar level (L_1) it begins to narrow progressively so that upon reaching the last lumbar (L_5) first sacral (S_1) interspace it has half of its original width. This ultimate narrow posterior ligamentous reinforcement contributes to an inherent structural weakness at the level where there is the greatest static stress and the greatest spinal movement producing the greatest kinetic strain (L_5-S_1). Further discussion of this will follow (Fig. 5).

Such is the anatomic construction of the anterior portion of the functional unit for its weight-bearing and shock-absorbing function. The anterior portion

6

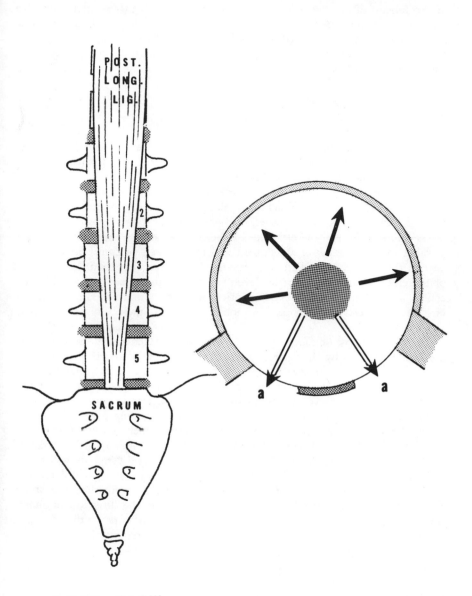

REAR VIEW

FIGURE 5. Diagrammatic sketch of posterior longitudinal ligamentous deficiency. The *rear view* drawing shows the narrowing of the ligament that begins at L₁. By the time it reaches L₅ it covers less than half the posterior disk margin. The double arrows in the small sketch show where disk herniation may bulge into the spinal canal.

of the functional unit is one of three "joints" contained in the total unit. The posterior portion of the functional unit containing the other two joints can now be discussed and incorporated into the total functional unit. In contrast to the anterior weight-bearing portion of the functional unit, the posterior portion has a guiding function.

Posterior Portion of Functional Unit

The posterior portion of the unit is composed of the two vertebral arches, two transverse processes, a central posterior spinous process, and paired articulations, inferior and superior, known as facets (Fig. 4).

The processes of the posterior arch, the transverse and the posterior spinous, are the points of muscular attachment. Because of the origin and insertion of muscles from one process to another, movement of the spine is possible. Because of the contractility and the elasticity of the muscles a large range of motion is possible and the manner of attachment and interspinous bridging provides balance of the *static* spine and strength for the *kinetic* spinal column. Maintenance of the erect posture is in part achieved by the sustained tonus of the muscles acting on these bony prominences. Motion and locomotion are also dependent on these muscles playing synchronously between their points of bony attachment.

The articulations, or facets, pilot the direction of movement between two adjacent vertebrae. By their directional planes they simultaneously prevent or restrict movement in a direction contrary to the planes of the articulation. They may be compared to the movement of wheels on railroad tracks in which forward and backward movement is possible but sideway movement is prevented.

The facets are arthrodial joints that function on a gliding basis. Lined with synovial tissue, they are separated by synovial fluid which is contained within an articular capsule. The plane of the facets, in their relation to the plane of the entire spine, determines the direction in which the two vertebrae will move. The direction, or plane, of the facets in any segment of the spine will determine the direction of movement permitted to that specific segment of the spine. The plane of the facets will simultaneously determine the direction of movement not permitted that spinal segment. Movement contrary to the direction of the plane obviously is prevented or, at least, markedly restricted.

Because in the lumbar region the facet planes lie in the vertical sagittal plane, they permit flexion and extension of the spine. Bending forwards and arching backwards are thus possible in the lumbar region. Due to the vertical sagittal facet plane, significant lateral bending and rotation are not possible. The male portion of the facets fitting into the female guiding portion permits movement in the direction of the guides, but lateral, oblique, or torque movement is mechanically prevented.

In the thoracic spine the facets are convex-concave and lie essentially in a horizontal plane. Movement permitted by this facet plane in the thoracic spine is lateral flexion, such as side bending and rotation about a vertical line. A combined movement of lateral flexion and rotation occurs here, for, in spinal

8

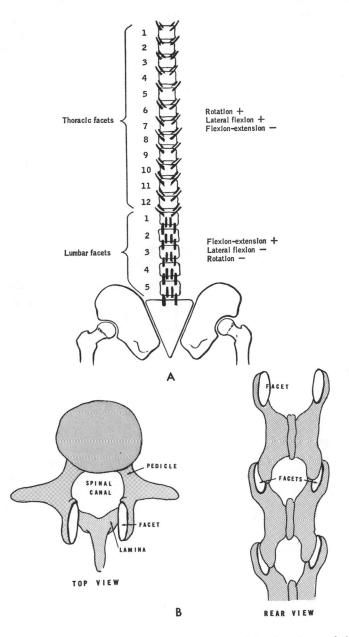

FIGURE 6. Direction of spinal movement is determined by the planes of the articular facets. A, The planes are vertical in the lumbar region thus only anterior-posterior motion (flexion-extension) is possible in this region. Lateral bending and rotation is prevented. The plane of the thoracic facets permits rotation and lateral flexion but denies flexion and extension. The direction of movement permitted and prevented are indicated for the individual sections. +, Indicates possible; −, prevented. B, Details showing facets.

column movement, no pure lateral bending is possible without some rotation and no true rotation is possible without some lateral flexion. Due to this facet plane, no significant flexion or extension movement in an anterior posterior plane is possible in the adult thoracic-spine segment (Fig. 6).

In brief, the direction of the facet plane that exists between two adjacent vertebrae in a functional unit determines the direction of movement of those two vertebrae. As the facets of the lumbar spine are vertical-sagittal in an anterior plane, movement of the lumbar spine exists in an anterior-posterior flexion-extension direction. The planes of the thoracic spine relegate to this segment all significant lateral flexion such as side bending and rotation of the total spine. All other significant movement is barred to these segments. In this generalization of total spinal movement the cervical spine segment is intentionally excluded.

TOTAL SPINE

The total vertebral column can now be visualized as the *sum total* of all the *functional units*, superimposed one upon the other, in an erect jointed column balanced against gravity and capable of movement. Having studied the functional anatomy of the individual functional unit we can now study the total vertebral column from a static and a kinetic viewpoint.

The *static* spine as observed from the side has three basic physiologic curves. A fourth curve, that of the coccyx below the sacral base, is a non-mobile inflexible curve with no pertinent effect upon man's attempt to maintain his balance in the erect position, and, therefore, its consideration is omitted in the study of the physiologic curves.

The entire spine is balanced on the sacrum, at its base, as a flexible segmented rod is balanced by a juggler. Immediately above the sacrum, the lowermost curve is the lumbar lordosis. This lordosis is convex anteriorly and forms its curve within a five vertebral body segment. The next curve, cephalad to the lumbar lordosis, is the thoracic curve which is termed the "dorsal kyphosis." The thoracic curve has its convexity posteriorly and being composed of 12 vertebrae has a curve of lesser curvature than is present in the lumbar curve. The bones of the thoracic vertebrae are smaller, and the disks are thinner, each disk being less pie-shaped than its comparative disk in the lumbar region. The cervical lordosis is the uppermost physiologic curve with an anterior convexity similar to the lumbar lordosis, and because of smaller vertebrae, thinner disks, and different bony configurations forms a smaller arc.

All three curves, the lumbar, the thoracic, and the cervical, in their ascent, must meet in a midline center of gravity to balance the weight distribution of the curve and to counter the eccentric loading of each curve. The side view of the three physiologic curves in the erect position may be considered as *posture* (Fig. 7).

The sacrum is the foundation platform upon which is balanced the superincumbent spinal column. As the sacrum is firmly attached to both ilia, these bones move en masse as one unit, constituting the pelvis. The pelvis is cen-

10

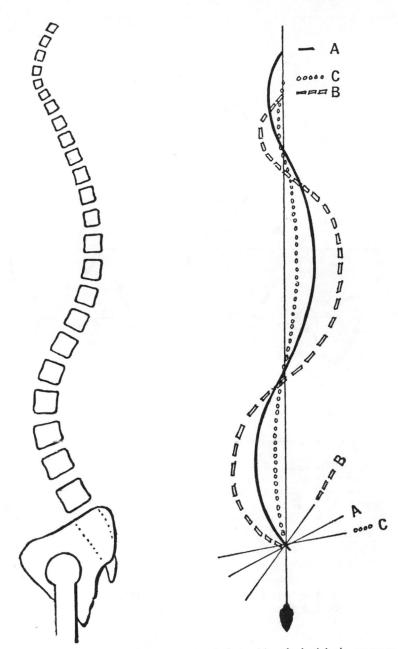

FIGURE 7. Static spine considered erect posture (relationship of physiologic curves to plumb line of gravity). Left, Lateral view of the upright spine with its static physiologic curves depicting posture. Right, The change in all superincumbent curves as influenced by change in the sacral base angle. All curves must be transected by the plumb line to remain gravity balanced. A, is physiologic; B, increased angle; and C, decreased sacral angle with flattened lumbar lordosis.

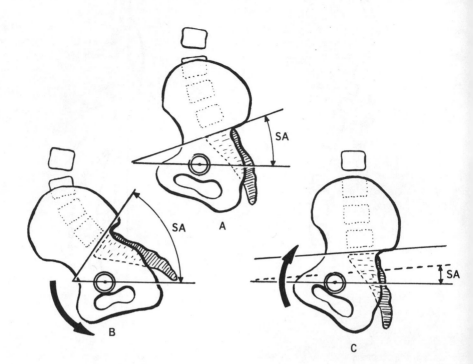

FIGURE 8. Sacral angle related to pelvic rotation. A, Pelvis is in a neutral position considered physiologic and the sacral angle (SA) is within the range of 30 degrees. B, Anterior depression of the pelvis rotates the sacrum and thus increases the angle to a more obtuse degree. C, Anterior elevation and posterior depression of the pelvis cause decrease of the sacral angle and consequently decrease the angle of take-off of the lumbar spine with decrease in the lumbar lordosis. This movement of the pelvis is clinically termed "tilting."

trally balanced on a transverse axis between two ball-bearing joints formed by the rounded femoral heads of the femors fitted into the cuplike acetabular sockets, which permit a rotatory motion in an anterior-posterior plane. By pivoting in a rotatory manner between these two lateral points, the pelvis may rotate back and forth, simultaneously rocking and changing the angle of the sacrum (Fig. 8).

Movement of the pelvis on its transverse axis constitutes "rotation" of the pelvis. Upward movement of the anterior pubic portion of the pelvis, termed "upward rotation," has the effect of lowering the sacrum with a decrease in the sacral angle. Downward movement of the front portion of the pelvis, called "tilting" of the pelvis, elevates the rear portion of the pelvis, changes the angle of the sacrum, and increases the sacral angle. The sacral angle is determined as

12

the line drawn parallel to the superior border of the sacrum measured in relationship to a horizontal line. The plane upon which the lumbar curve is balanced and ascends is thus variable and can change in its inclination according to the relationship of the pelvis.

As the lumbar spine ascends upwards at an angle perpendicular to the level of the sacral surface, the acute angle of the sacrum causes the lumbar spine to arise at a slight vertical angle. Thus the lumbar spine needs only a slight degree of arching to return to midline. With an increase in the sacral angle, due to tilting of the pelvis, the plane of the sacrum becomes more obtuse, the lumbar spine takes off at a sharper angle to the horizontal and must, therefore, arc through a sharper curve to return to midline. The greater the sacral angle the more-angled the lumbar take-off demands that the curve which will bring the spine back into center of gravity balance must be even sharper. Those few words, "the greater must be the curve," specify essentially a greater *lordosis* of the lumbar spine.

In contrast a smaller angle brought about by elevating the pubic bone which depresses the sacrum, thereby decreasing the angle of the sacral base, permits a more erect lumbar spine with a smaller arc, or lordosis. This movement of the pelvis is called *tilting** and the effect on the lumbar lordosis termed *flattening*.

As the pelvic angle determines the angle of lumbar take-off and influences the degree of lumbar curvature so must the degree of lumbar lordosis influence the degree of the superincumbent thoracic curve. The return to mid-line to prevent eccentric loading will always force a flexible vertical balanced rod to curve back towards the mid-line. As there is insignificant anterior-posterior flexion-extension mobility of the thoracic spine, balance occurs as a rigid total segment moving at the thoraco-lumbar joint to maintain its equilibrium (T_{12}-L_1). At the summit, the balance of the remaining spine is achieved in the cervical region which balances the head and keeps it at the center of gravity.

The three physiologic curves that comprise the *static* spine and designate *posture* are unequivocally influenced by the sacral angle. In other words, pelvic rotation is the mainstay of erect posture. Lateral viewing of the three curves of the non-moving erect spine gives a true picture of the posture of the erect *adult*.

While one quarter of the adult spine is composed of disk material, the remaining three quarters consists of bony vertebrae. As the upper and lower vertebral cartilaginous plates are essentially parallel, the degree of curving is largely determined by the shape of the disks. If all the vertebrae were superimposed on each other without the interposition of the intervertebral disks, the physiologic postural curves would not exist. The disk-less spine would form a very slight curve with its convexity posterior. The curve formed by the disk-less spine would resemble that of the newborn child. Development of the upright adult posture evolves in a chronological pattern from the first posture of the newborn.

---

*"Tilting" (here employed to mean "to cause flattening of the lumbar lordosis") is used in a clinical sense, whereas functional anatomists use the term in an opposite sense of the word to imply anterior elevation of the pelvis.

The spine of the newborn has none of the adult physiologic curves, but instead has a total flexion curve of the curled up infant *in utero* position. The total curve is slightly more arched than is the ultimate adult thoracic kyphotic curve, and the curve is of similar convexity. There are no lordotic curves in the lumbar or cervical spinal areas of the newborn child.

During the first six to eight weeks of life the child raises his head and by this antigravity maneuver initiates the muscular action of the erector muscles that form the cervical lordosis. As crawling and sitting ultimately evolve, the lower lumbar spinal curve develops in an antigravity action. The dorsal kyphosis has no antigravity influence even when an erect posture is reached, so that the change that evolves is merely a slight increase in its initial *in utero* convexity.

The addition of the two lordotic curves gives primarily the antigravity effect of the erector muscles which develop in the child as it attempts and finally achieves the upright-erect position. The lordotic curves originate partly from the original strength of the antigravity muscle and in some measure from the weakness of the opposite musculature, such as that which exists in the abdominal muscle and in the anterior neck-flexor muscles.

The lumbar lordosis is caused largely by the failure of the hip flexors to stretch and elongate. In the fetal position the hips and knees are flexed against the abdomen of the child in its "curled up in a ball" position. As the legs extend, the iliopsoas muscle elongates slowly but incompletely. The iliacus because of its influence upon the inner aspect of the ilium to the anterior-upper thigh acts to keep the hips flexed. The psoas originates from the anterior aspect of the lumbar spine and enters upon the anterior aspect of the femur. As the hips extend to assume the erect posture, extension at the hip joints causes a simultaneous forward traction on the lumbar spine via the psoas attachment, causing anterior convexity or lordosis (Fig. 9).

POSTURE

The upright adult exhibits balanced physiologic curves. Static spinal configuration can be considered "good posture" if it is an effortless, non-fatiguing posture, painless to the individual who can remain erect for reasonable periods of time, and present an aesthetically acceptable appearance.

These criteria of normalcy must be considered in ascertaining the cause of painful states and the factors demanding correction. Significant deviations from physiologic static spinal curves can cause discomfort and disability.

There are many factors that influence adult posture but there are three factors that supersede all others in their prevalence and frequency: (1) Familial-hereditary postures, such as marked dorsal kyphotic spine, a noticeable "sway back," etc.; variations in ligamentous laxity, muscle tone, and even psychologic motor drive have a familial-hereditary component. (2) Structural abnormalities influence posture. Such abnormalities may be congenital or acquired, may be skeletal, muscular, or neurologic, and may be static or progressive. Postural defects can occur as the result of neuromuscular diseases, such as cerebral palsy, parkinsonism, and hemiplegia. The influence on the postural structures from

14

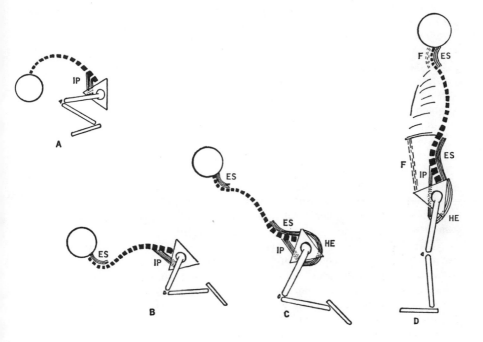

FIGURE 9. Chronologic development of posture. A, The total curve of the fetal spine *in utero*. B, Formation of the cervical lordosis when the head overcomes gravity. C, Formation of the second lordotic (lumbar) curve due to the antigravity force of the lumbar erector spinae (ES) muscles and the restriction of the iliopsoas muscles (IP). D, Erect adult posture showing the strong antigravity erector muscles (ES and HE hip extensors) and the weak flexor (F) muscles of the neck and abdomen.

diseases, such as rheumatoid arthritis and poliomyelitis, and from peripheral nerve injuries needs no elaboration. More insidious in its influence and admittedly more controversial in its acceptance is (3) the posture of habit and training.

Postural influences attributable to a familial or hereditary origin and postural deviations established by the external influences of neuromuscular, articular, or bony pathology can usually be established by correct history, complete physical examination, and specific laboratory and roentgen-ray studies. Many diseases portray a specific diagnostic picture that reveals the diagnosis at a glance. The influence of some diseases on posture may be less clearly defined, but further study of the effect of disease on posture can produce additional diagnostic tools.

The effects of habit or training on posture presents a study that has its own share of controversy and difference of opinion. Postural training in childhood by parental control or training by educators in our schools has a profound influence in laying the groundwork of ultimate adult posture. Posture is to a large degree habit and from training and repetition can become a subconscious habit. The subconscious habit of posture is manifested not only in static posture but to a large degree in kinetic patterns. Repetition of faulty action can result in faulty kinetic function and repeated faulty posture patterns can become ingrained.

Posture must also be viewed from the cultural aspects of training, background, and childhood environment. Parental example is of undoubted significance in the establishment of accepted normal posture. Competition and example from siblings or classmates will also leave its mark on the psyche which in turn molds the postural patterns.

Posture to a large degree is also a somatic depiction of the inner emotions. There is no doubt that posture can be considered a somatization of the psyche. We stand and we move as we feel. Our stance and our movements mirror clearly to the observer our psychologic inner drives or their absence. Consciously or unconsciously we assume a pose to portray our inner feelings, and we move in a manner that depicts our attitude toward ourselves, our fellow man, and our environment. Our posture is "organ language," a feeling-expression, in fact a postural exteriorization of our inner feelings.

The depressed, dejected person will stand in a "drooped" postural manner with the upper back rounded and the shoulders depressed by the "weight of the world carried on his back." This is the familiar bodily expression when one is too tired to "stand any more of this." Such posture is a picture of fatigue and becomes in itself a fatiguing posture. The posture of fatigue places a chronic ligamentous strain upon an individual and the muscular effort exerted to relieve the strain may be too feeble to be effectual.

The hyperactive hyperkinetic person will portray his feelings in posture as well as in the abruptness and irregularity of his movements. The movements of alertness need not be, and, in fact usually are not, those of efficiency and effectiveness. This posture depicts that of the uneasy aggressor, in combat pose, ready to leap or ready to withdraw in a defensive crouch. In observing this type of person, the doctor need not ask his psychologic attitude but should merely observe his sitting, standing, walking, response to questions, and movements during the interview and examination.

The tall girl may stand slumped. In childhood she wished to be shorter as were her companions. She stooped "down to their height." Her counterpart, the short girl, stood "to her full height" to be taller, by standing on her toes, with her head erect, her chest protruding and her low back arched. The full-bosomed girl, influenced by teasing or fearing to lack modesty, sat, stood, and walked with rounded shoulders to decrease the apparent size of her bosom.

All patterns of posture assumed in childhood for real or imagined results form a pattern that becomes deep seated. The pattern becomes not only a psychic pattern, but it gradually molds the tissues into somatic patterns that remain a structural monument to early psychic molding. When the age of "reason" or realization is reached the posture is largely fixed in its structural composition and is deeply established in the subconscious. Without extreme persistent effort to change, that posture will become a permanent fixture.

16

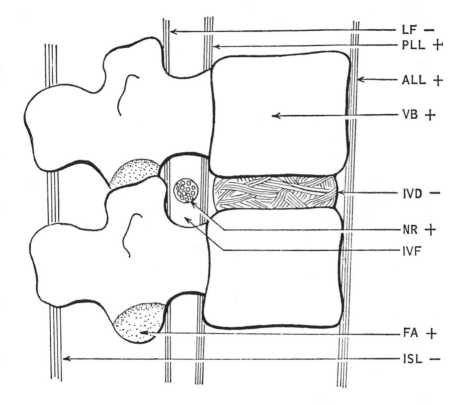

FIGURE 10. Pain-sensitive tissues of the functional unit. The tissues labelled + are pain sensitive in that they contain sensory nerve endings that are capable of causing pain when irritated. Tissues labelled — are devoid of sensory nerve endings.

IVF = Intervertebral foramen containing nerve root (NR).
LF   = Ligamentum flavum
PLL = Posterior longitudinal ligament
ALL = Anterior longitudinal ligament
IVD = Annulus fibrosus of intervertebral disk
FA   = Facet articular cartilage
ISL = Interspinous ligament

Patterns depicting the picture of inner feeling can be acquired in later life. The tired depressed patient will enter the doctor's office walking "as he feels" and in a manner that will make it obvious to everyone "the way he feels." A patient may even hope to gain sympathy in this way. The manner of answering questions fortifies the impression garnered by the observation of posture and gait. The tone is flat and the speech without inflection. The handshake is limp, weak, tired, and unenthusiastic. The unfortunate aspect of this type of patient

17

is the active adherence and perseverance to his state of mind that will rebel against the prescribed treatment for the diagnosed postural problem. No active sustained effort on the part of the patient can be hoped for.

On the other hand, the hyperactive over-reacting patient with his "bone-crushing pump-handle" handshake is not difficult to evaluate. The erratic and uncoordinated muscular activity of this individual not infrequently leads to unnecessary and excessive efforts, but the joints and ligaments are unprepared for the abrupt, erratic movement that ensues and dysfunction results.

The pain-causing postural pattern can be ascertained by understanding the deviation from what is considered normal. A full evaluation of the mechanisms of pain production in the *static* then in the *kinetic* spines will follow, but the exact sites of pain production must first be determined. When the site of tissue capable of eliciting pain can be located, the specific movement or positions of the vertebral components that irritate these tissues can be established. For the evaluation of the sites in the vertebral column capable of painful reaction we must return to the *functional unit* (Fig. 10).

TISSUE SITES OF PAIN ORIGIN

The intervertebral disk itself is a non-pain-sensitive tissue. The total disk is an inert tissue and the nucleus has been found completely free of any sensory type of nerve endings. Nerve endings have been found in the annulus, but neurophysiologic studies have failed to discover pain sensory transmission from these nerves. The disks, therefore, both annulus and nucleus, must be considered insensitive to pain sensations.

If the absence of sensory nerves emanating from the disk be accepted it must be assumed that it is not possible to consider the disk a pain-producing unit. The commonplace disk-pain must, therefore, originate from contiguous tissues, with the disk itself in some manner participating in the instigation of disk-pain by its action on these surrounding tissues.

If the internal pressure within a normal disk is experimentally increased by injecting saline solution into the disk the mere increase of such pressure does not cause pain. In a disk, however, that has previously been degenerated, which degeneration can be considered fragmentation of the annulus with a dehydrated nucleus, increase in the interdiskal pressure causes an ache in the region of the low back.

If the same method of increasing pressure within a disk of known degeneration is used no pain sensation occurs when the posterior longitudinal ligament is anesthetized by procaine. It can be assumed then that the irritation of the posterior longitudinal ligament by increase in internal pressure within a degenerated disk is the mechanism of pain production, and the posterior longitudinal ligament is the pain-sensitive tissue. The posterior longitudinal ligament therefore must contain sensory nerve endings.

It is apparent that a normal disk has sufficient elasticity and resiliency to withstand significant increases in internal pressure which will prevent a bulging irritation of contiguous tissues. Degeneration of a disk due to annular fragmentation decreases its resiliency and resistance to increase in internal pressure permitting encroachment on surrounding tissues.

The ligamentum flavum and the interspinous ligaments are non-sensitive. Similarly, stimulation or movement of the dura mater elicits no sensation of pain. These tissues, therefore, must be classified as insensitive to pain.

The synovial lining of the facets and the articular capsule of these joints are richly supplied by sensory as well as vasomotor nerves. The synovial tissues of these joint spaces respond to stimuli and inflammations as do all other synovial joint tissues elsewhere in the body. Inflammatory responses of these tissues result in swelling and engorgement of the synovial linings, increase viscosity of the synovial fluid, causing periarticular muscle spasm that results in progressive limitation of movement. The part becomes "frozen" or at least significantly immobilized. Inflammation of synovial joints produces dull to severe pain depending on the severity and extent of the inflammation.

The concomitant muscle spasm that accompanies spine dysfunction is in itself capable of eliciting pain. In animal experiments, painful irritation of the lumbosacral joints and ligaments causes reflex spasm of the erector spinae and hamstring muscles. This spasm in a human being undoubtedly is painful. In addition to pain resulting from the joint and ligamentous irritation, there can arise irritation from the sustained muscle spasm, compression of the interposed intervertebral disk by the spasm of the muscle, which will result in pain if any disk degeneration exists. In the presence of any disk degeneration the spasm can constitute a significant compressive force. Multiple factors, such as these, can be seen to contribute to the production of pain at the functional unit level.

Another factor is the sciatic nerve root which emerges through the intervertebral foramen. It is a combined motor-sensory nerve and thus is a pain-sensitive nerve. Irritation of this nerve evokes pain localized to the dermatome distribution of the specific rootlet irritated. Mere contact with the nerve root is enough to cause pain. Although traction on the nerve has been claimed as the necessary irritant for causing pain, such is not the case. Merely touching without *stretching* the nerve will cause pain. The obvious verification of this is obtained in the fact that the lumbar nerve roots have considerable freedom of movement and, therefore, traction upon these nerve roots would be exceedingly difficult.

We have ascertained which tissues within the functional unit are capable of eliciting pain, and we have depicted the static erect spine by combining and superimposing the functional units. Now we must make our upright person move and, in moving, the normal must be established so that deviations capable of causing pain can be understood.

KINETIC ASPECT OF TOTAL SPINE

The total erect spine that has been described in its static postural state is capable of movement and now must be analyzed in its kinetic potentialities. The functional units are the component operational units of the entire spinal column and, as the units individually move, so moves the total column.

Movement is initiated by muscular action exerting its traction effect through its muscular attachments upon the bony prominences of the functional unit. A constant attempt is made by the antigravity forces to maintain balance against gravity. Of these antigravity forces, muscular action initiated by a proprioceptively stimulated righting reflex immediately attempts to correct the "off-center" shift. During movement, the body makes a constant effort to maintain its balance.

.Movement of the total spine has been previously pictured as that of an articulated flexible rod requiring movement at each component segment. Movement at the anterior portion of the functional unit is permitted by the fluid shift of the nucleus pulposus within its elastic annulus. Excessive movement is prevented by the longitudinal ligaments which, by their resiliency, exert a cushioning effect and thus protect the fibers of the annulus from bearing the full tearing effect of forceful flexion or excessive extension.

The facets have been ascribed as the guiding portion of the functional unit permitting flexion-extension in the lumbar region and rotation lateral-flexion in the thoracic area because of the directional plane of the facet joints. All movement contrary to this articular plane is essentially prevented.

The extent of the permitted range of motion is thus determined by the extensibility of the longitudinal ligaments, the elasticity of the articular capsule, the fluidity of the disk, and the elasticity of the muscles. Since it is known that direction of movement of the lumbar spine is the effect of flexion and extension, it may be asked to what extent these movements are possible in the normal spine.

Extension of the lumbar spine may be slight, but it is usually possible to a moderate degree. Most children have the capability of arching backwards to a large degree, and with training and persistent exercise this function may persist through adulthood. Inherited ligamentous laxity will enhance this more extreme hyperextension. The anterior longitudinal ligament plays the major restricting role in limiting hyperextension.

Forward flexion of the lumbar spine is possible to a much smaller extent than is extension. Such forward flexion of the lumbar spine is possible *only* to the *extent of and slightly more* than the *reversal* of the static lumbar *lordosis* (Fig. 11).

The lumbar spine, which is usually composed of five vertebrae, must have its movement occur within the five intervertebral interspaces. In total flexion the degree of flexion movement varies at each interspace. Most forward flexion movement occurs at the last interspace which is the intervertebral space between the last lumbar (L_5) and the sacrum (S_1). An estimated three quarters (75 per cent) of all lumbar flexion occurs at this interspace, which marks the junction of the lumbar spine to the sacral-pelvic bone and constitutes the *lumbosacral joint*.

Owing to the absence of flexion in the thoracic spine and with the postulation that 75 per cent of lumbar flexion occurs at the lumbosacral joint, it may be argued then that 75 per cent of all spine flexion occurs at the lumbosacral joint.

The remaining percentage of forward flexion is proportioned between the

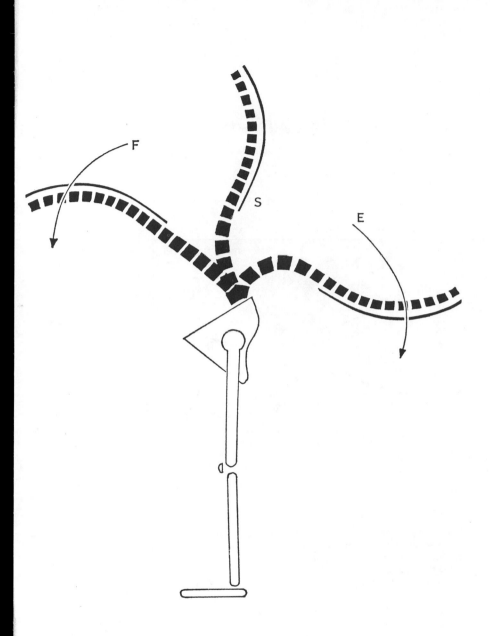

FIGURE 11.   Flexion-extension of total spine. Composite diagram depicting flexion and extension of total spine. Flexion of the lumbar spine occurs to the extent of reversing slightly past the lordosis whereas extension is moderate. In all movements of flexion, extension, or static erect position the thoracic spine does not alter its curve. (F = flexion; S = static spine; E = extension.)

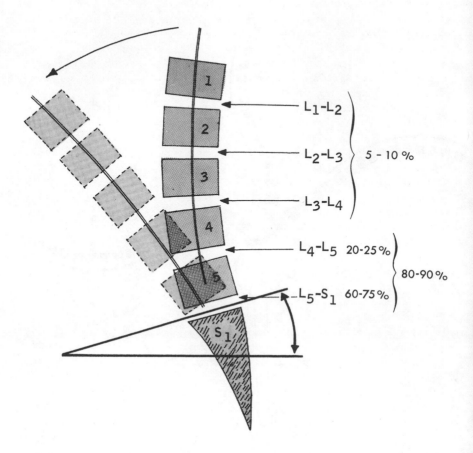

FIGURE 12. Segmental site and degree of lumbar spine flexion. The degree of flexion noted in the lumbar spine as a percentage of total spine flexion is indicated. The major portion of flexion (75 per cent) occurs at the lumbosacral joint, 20 to 25 per cent of flexion occurs at L_4-L_5 interspace, and the remainder 5 to 10 per cent distributed between L_1-L_4. The forward flexed diagram indicates the mere reversal past lordosis of total flexion of the lumbar curve.

remainder of the lumbar-vertebral interspaces. Approximately 20 per cent of flexion occurs between L_4 and L_5 vertebrae, and the remaining 5 or 10 per cent occurs between L_1 and L_4. The greatest portion of this last 5 to 10 per cent of flexion is found between L_2 to L_4 (Fig. 12).

The theory of *total* trunk *flexion* may be summarized as occurring primarily at the lumbosacral joint and to a lesser degree between the remainder of the lumbar vertebrae with total lumbar flexion limited to the extent of reversal of the static lordosis. Extension of the total spinal column also occurs exclusively within the lumbar segment but to a greater degree than the extent of flexion. No significant flexion-extension occurs in the dorsal spine.

If a person were to bend forward in an attempt to touch his fingers to the floor without bending at the knees, he would require more than the degree of flexion attributed to the lumbar spine flexion. Were this lumbar curve reversal the only flexion possible for the individual, less than half the distance towards the floor would be reached. Additional bending must be possible, and this flexion occurs at the hip joints.

The flexion possible at the hips is attributed to rotation of the pelvis around the fulcrum of the two lateral hip joints. Such rotation occurs in an anterior-posterior sagittal plane with the anterior portion or symphysis pubis area lowering or rising, while the sacrum at the posterior end of the rocker describes the same arc. The level of the sacrum changes its angle in respect to the horizontal as does a balanced teeter board.

As the pelvis rotates forward, the sacral angle becomes more obtuse, and the lumbar spines takes off at a more forward ascent. If no flexion of the lumbar spine had taken place when full forward rotation of the pelvis had occurred, the person may have been able to bend forward to a significant degree with his fingers almost touching the floor if his hips were sufficiently limber to permit that degree of pelvic rotation.

Smooth symmetrical total-bending, however, is the result of the physiologic manner in which man is intended to bend. This is done with pelvic rotation and flexion of the spine occurring simultaneously. A smooth-graded ratio must exist between the degree of pelvic rotation and the degree of lumbar lordotic reversal that constitutes the *lumbar-pelvic rhythm*. The mathematical relationship of lumbar curve, or the lordosis, and reversal to the simultaneous degree of rotation of the pelvis, which is the change in the sacral angle, constitutes the fundamental *kinetic* concept of the spine. This rhythmic relationship of spine-trunk-flexion to pelvic rotation is similar in body mechanics to the *scapulo-humeral rhythm* considered to be the physiologic *kinetic* pattern of the shoulder girdle.

LUMBAR-PELVIC RHYTHM

The lumbar-pelvic rhythm (Fig. 13) can be perceived as the ratio between two movements occurring simultaneously in one plane. Reversal of the lumbar curve is difficult to grade in a numerical formula that would be simple, clear, and concise. The *lumbar* portion of the rhythm is initially a flattening, then a gradual reversal of an arc that was not originally a perfect sphere. The lumbar curve does not reverse equally at all points along its sphere. The difference of movement at the L_5-S_1 segment compared to the movement between L_2-L_3 indicates the irregularity of the arc as it flattens out and reverses. Nevertheless, there is significant smoothness of curve change to correlate it in a smooth kinetic relationship with a simultaneous secondary movement of pelvic rotation.

During the change of lumbar curve from concave to flat, to convex, occurs the secondary movement of pelvic rotation. The *pelvic* phase of the rhythm is merely the ¬otation of the pelvis around the transverse axis of the two hip joints. Pelvic rotation, in total spinal flexion, is rotation of the pelvis starting with the sacral angle as noted in the *static* spine, followed by a smooth gradual increase of the angle as the anterior portion of the pelvis descends and the posterior aspect ascends. The sacral angle which increases in flexion decreases in extension as the body returns to the erect *static* stance. The grading of this

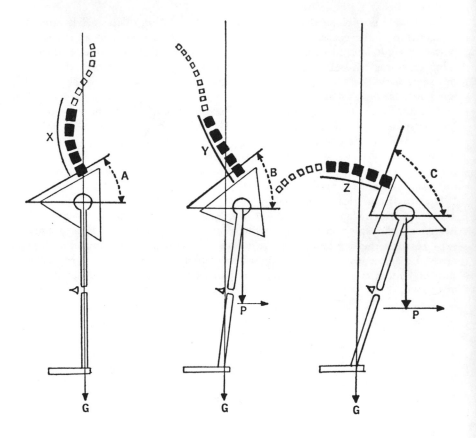

FIGURE 13. Lumbar-pelvic rhythm of total flexion. Left, Static spine in upright position with postural lumbar lordosis (X) arising from lumbosacral angle (A). The posture is balanced plumb line through the hip joints. Center, Beginning flexion with early reversal of lordotic curve (Y), simultaneous rotation of pelvis with increase in LSA to B and posterior shift of center of gravity (P). Thoracic spine moves with no change in its curvature. Right, Total flexion reveals that the lumbar spine has flexed past degree (Z) of lumbar flattening, pelvic rotation has fully rotated around the hip joint (C) and the hips are further posterior to plumb-line center of gravity to maintain balance. Thoracic spine remains unchanged.

rotation is easy to calibrate mathematically as the movement consists merely of rotation around a central point.

Lumbar-pelvic rhythm is a simultaneous movement in a rhythmic ratio of a lumbar movement to a pelvic rotation, the sum-total-movement consisting in the person's bending forward and returning to an erect position. At any phase of total body flexion the extent of lumbar curve flattening must be accompanied by a proportionate degree of pelvic rotation. When complete body flexion has been attained, the lumbar curve must have fully straightened and reversed, thus presenting a lumbar convexity while the pelvis must have rotated to the full extent permitted by the hip joints. The rhythm is so smooth and precise that at every point in the process, there will be equality between lumbar reversal and pelvic rotation.

A related phase of the lumbar-pelvic rhythm which must occur simultaneously (although it cannot be computed in the basic rhythm) is that of forward and backward shifting of the hips along a horizontal plane. In such movement the hips move anteriorly and posteriorly to the center of gravity. During forward flexion of the total trunk a shift backwards occurs, but upon returning to the erect static stance the trunk shifts forward. This anterior-posterior shift of the pelvic fulcrum is a readjustment of superincumbent weight over a center of gravity. If the hips fail to center and adjust properly, forward flexion would place the body off balance, and it would fall forward. The shift of the pelvic fulcrum point again balances an equal weight distribution ahead of and behind the weight-bearing point of the feet. This must occur to permit the *lumbar-pelvic* phases of the rhythm to operate; otherwise, the eccentric superincumbent weight impedes synchronous flexion and extension. The anterior-posterior shift thus is an integral part of the *pelvic* portion of the *lumbar-pelvic rhythm* even though it is not mathematically computed and included in the basic L-P rhythm.

In the discussion of the lumbar-pelvic rhythm the emphasis has been on *flexion*, but the exact converse of the rhythm must occur in the return to erect position after flexion. It is obvious that return from any point must begin at a concise point in the rhythm at some place during the descent. Just as every point in the lumbar flexion must be matched by a concise point in the degree of pelvic rotational tilting so must return to the erect be synchronously perfect. Full return to upright finds the pelvis derotated to its more acute lumbosacral angle while the lumbar curve resumes its erect static lordosis (Fig. 13 in reverse).

Man in his action of bending forwards and straightening up must conform to accurate smooth lumbar-pelvic rhythm which, being kinetic, is a neuromuscular pattern of action as well as a mechanical function. This neuromuscular pattern is partly acquired and partly inherited. Deviation, however, can occur, and faulty habit can be learned and repeated until the deviation becomes a deep-seated habit pattern. Proper rhythm similarly can be perfected by learning and acquired habits.

The neuromuscular pattern must be precise and work together with faultless mechanical action of the spine. All the moving parts must be unimpeded. As any defective part in an otherwise integrated machine will impair total function so will inadequacy of any of the component parts of the lumbar-pelvic mechanism destroy proper rhythm.

Reference to component parts again draws attention to the functional unit. Adequacy of the unit demands competent disks. Anatomically symmetrical facets are necessary to permit accurate gliding, and the synovial linings of the articular surfaces must present no impediment to smooth motion.

The longitudinal ligaments the main function of which is limitation of motion must in turn permit sufficient and free movement existing throughout the length of the ligament. Segmental limitation in the elongation of any one ligament would cause excessive movement in the other less restricted segments. Limited elongation of the entire length of the longitudinal ligament would totally impair the lumbar phase of the rhythm. Physiologic spine flexion requires resiliency for the posterior longitudinal ligament while the paraspinous muscles must have equal elasticity.

Pelvic rotation is directly dependent on the adequacy of the hip joints to rotate fully in a ball-bearing manner. This requires a normal hip-joint socket working bilaterally. The intactness of the joint socket must be accompanied by resilient periarticular tissues and good muscular control of hip function. The third phase of the lumbar-pelvic rhythm in which the pelvic joint alters its relationship to the center of gravity also demands symmetrical integrity of the hip joints.

LIGAMENTOUS-MUSCULAR SUPPORT

Consideration of the periarticular tissues and muscular influence on the kinetic spine involves once again a discussion of the static spine because a balanced erect static spine requires minimal muscular effort.

Physiologic erect balance is essentially a ligamentous function relieved by intermittent small muscular contractions that are triggered by proprioceptive reflexes of the joints and ligaments. The muscles of an erect but relaxed man are electromyographically silent except for those in the gastrocnemius groups. The calf muscles which balance the leg at the ankle joint are the only continually active muscular group affecting posture.

Ligamentous support is effortless and thus not fatiguing. Excessive or prolonged ligamentous stress is relieved by muscular contraction and, as muscular effort is fatiguing, is held to a minimum for economy of energy expenditure. Good posture requires balance between ligamentous support and minimal, yet adequate, muscle tone. Improper posture or prolonged stress from awkward positions causes protracted ligamentous strain resulting in discomfort. Strain may arise because of muscular fatigue which no longer affords ligamentous relief.

For proper posture, the static spine is dependent on the pelvic angle. The pelvis is held in ligamentous balance by the anterior hip joint and the "Y" ligament. This "Y" ligament, the iliopectineal ligament, is a fibrous reinforcement of the anterior portion of the hip joint that prevents hyperextension of the hip. In erect stance, man "leans forward on this ligament."

26

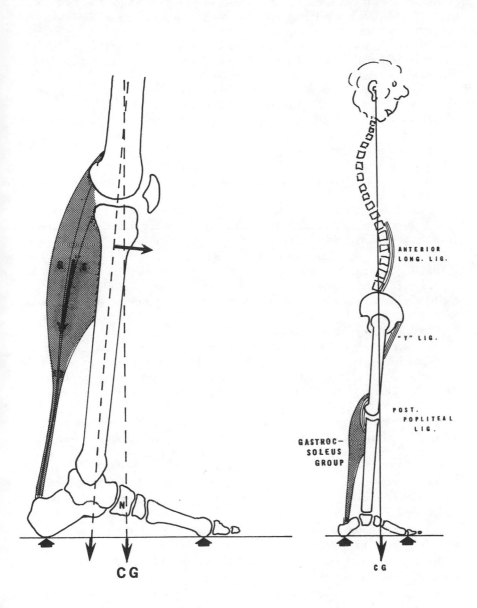

FIGURE 14. Static spine support. The relaxed person leans on his ligaments: the ileofemoral ligament, ("Y" ligament of Bigelow), the anterior longitudinal ligament, and the posterior knee ligaments. The ankle cannot be "locked," but by leaning forward only a few degrees the gastrocnemius must contract to support the entire body. Relaxed erect posture is principally ligamentous with only the gastroc-soleus muscle group active.

The knee joint can similarly be "locked" in extension when it relies on the posterior popliteal tissue that prevents over-extending the knees. This position eliminates the need for any muscular effort on the part of the quadriceps femoris. The lumbar spine can "lean" on the anterior-longitudinal ligament and the abdominal wall. The ankle joint, however, cannot be "locked" in any position so that muscular effort is required constantly.

The pelvis is further supported by the tensor fascia latae. These fascial bands mechanically assist the "Y" ligaments as well as limit lateral shift of the pelvis. Their course from the iliac crests downwards and backwards to insert at the iliotibial band at the knee lends itself well to reinforcing the "Y" ligament and helps lock the knee (Fig. 14).

The pelvic angle is the key to ligamentous posture. Rotation of the pelvis will initiate a total unlocking of all the balancing joints and necessitate muscular effort.

To study the erect person functioning in anterior-posterior plane, it is best to view him from the rear because it will then be possible to see the deviations from the normal in their relation to an imaginary vertical line.

The upright supporting beams of the pelvic floor are the legs, and if the parallel legs are equal in length the supported platform will be horizontal. If the tibia and femurs of both legs are in direct alignment and of equal length, the femoral heads must be equidistant from the ground, and the transverse axis through the femoral heads must be horizontal. Balanced between these two points the pelvis will rotate around a level axis.

In the static spine a level pelvis viewed from behind will reveal the spine ascending from the pelvic base at right angles and so continuing cephalad will find the head perched in direct mid-line over the center of the sacral point (Fig. 15). This head-pelvic center relationship obviously presupposes a straight spine.

A structurally straight spine of adequate flexibility will permit symmetrical bilateral side-bending. When we recall that lateral spine movement occurs in the thoracic region and not in the lumbar area, an equal degree of bending to the left or to the right will demand that the mid-point be level. This action requires a truly vertical lumbar spine. Symmetry in the act of side-bending requires lateral flexibility of the spine. As no significant lateral bending occurs in the lumbar spine the angle of take-off from the lumbar spine at the pelvic level will determine the amount of correction the dorsal spine must take to effect a return to the center of gravity.

Another important factor is leg-length discrepancy which will cause a pelvic obliquity. The causes of leg-length differences are numerous. A unilateral *genu valgum* or unilateral *genu recurvatum* will cause the side involved to be of shorter length. A unilateral leg-length discrepancy can result from fractures, articular disease, amputation *per se* or from an improperly fitted prosthesis. Childhood diseases (such as osteochondrosis, poliomyelitis, and hip dysplasia), that may impair unilateral leg growth, can lead to unequal leg lengths in adult life. The effect of leg-length difference on the pelvic level has an apparent influence on the static spine when it is seen from the anterior-posterior position, and the obliquity of the pelvis has an equal effect on the kinetic spine.

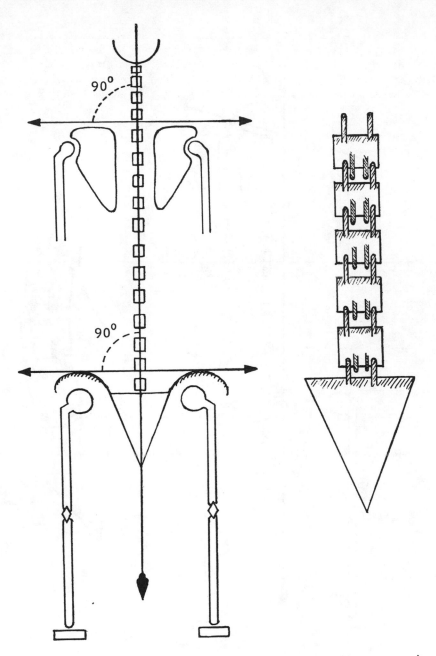

FIGURE 15. Spinal alignment from anterior-posterior aspect. Anterior-posterior view of the erect human spine. With both legs equal in length the spine supports the pelvis in a level horizontal plane and the spine, taking off at a right (90 degree) angle, ascends in a straight line. The facets shown in the enlarged drawing on the right show their parallel alignment and proper symmetry in this erect position.

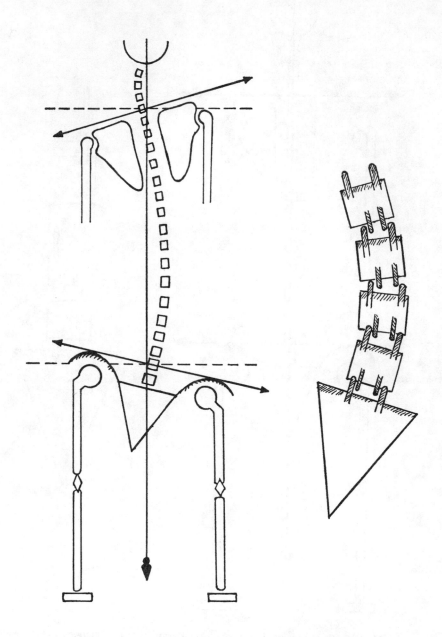

FIGURE 16. Pelvic obliquity and its relationship to spinal alignment. Anterior view of an oblique pelvis due to a leg-length discrepancy. Owing to pelvic slant in a lateral plane the spinal take-off is at a lateral angle. The flexible spine will curve in an attempt to compensate and the facets of the curving spine will become asymmetrical in relationship to each other.

FACET PLANES

In the lumbar spine the facets are vertically parallel and their proper alignment demands a straight line. A curve in the lumbar spine will displace the relationship of the facets. The spinal curve of the structural scoliosis portrays vividly this imbalance. A curvature similar to this structural scoliosis may exist merely because an otherwise flexible spine is affected by a pelvic obliquity caused by differential in leg length.

When the spine is straight and the facets symmetrical the articular surfaces glide without friction. If the facets deviate in their direction of movement, the articulating surfaces are no longer parallel, and friction or impingement may occur at some point in the glide (Fig. 16). In this respect the scoliosis resulting from a short leg does not differ markedly from a structural scoliosis.

Unilateral impairment of movement of any of the joints participating in the total movement of the lumbar-pelvic rhythm can cause asymmetry in flexion or extension. A hip joint that is damaged and will not rotate fully will prevent full rotation of the pelvis around its axis. Axis rotation is hindered at one end of its bilateral supports. One of the pair of ball-bearing joints "binds" in its rotation and thus places excessive strain at the other end. An extra-articular restriction of the joint, such as tight hamstrings on one side, can cause a similar asymmetrical restriction. The *lumbar-pelvic rhythm* becomes impeded by a unilateral defective part and the two halves of the body, left and right, perform the rhythm unequally. Furthermore, a fused ankle, by impeding the third phase of the rhythm, the posterior shift of the pelvis, has its adverse influence on the total rhythmic cycle.

Intrinsic structural facet asymmetry within an otherwise straight spine can adversely influence the rhythm. This asymmetry must be confirmed by x-ray studies and cannot be determined exclusively on clinical observation. As the total pelvic-lumbar rhythm mechanism requires all the component parts to function without hindrance, any break in continuity, any "weak link in the chain," will ultimately result in over-all stress and the eventual breakdown of pain-free motion.

SUMMARY

The human spine is an articulated flexible structure composed of superimposed *functional units*; it is clear then that the total function of the spine depends on the integrity of each component part. The total functional unit is divided into two segments. The anterior portion is a hydraulic weight-bearing shock-absorbing structure composed of two vertebrae and their interposed disk. The posterior section contains the articulating facets and functions as a guiding mechanism without weight-bearing facets.

The total spine comprises three physiologic curves which are formed by the shape of the intervening disk and in the lumbar segment forms a "lordosis," in the dorsal spine a "kyphosis," and in the cervical spine another "lordosis."

These three curves transect the plumb line of gravity in order to remain in a state of balance.

Because the plane of the facets directs the movement of the spine at each segment, movement in a direction contrary to the facet plane is prevented. Vertical position of the lumbar facets determines anterior-posterior movement in a sagittal direction. Horizontal concave articular placement in the thoracic spinal segment places lateral bending and rotation of the total spine at this section.

The entire spine is balanced on an undulating pelvic base. The sacral portion of the pelvis by changing angle influences the superincumbent curves and thereby determines the *static* posture. Static stance is a ligamentously supported position requiring minimal muscular action.

The *kinetic* spine flexes and extends in a pattern of *lumbar-pelvic rhythm*. Smooth movement of the rhythm demands good neuromuscular integration, adequate flexibility of tissues, and competence of the participating joints.

Pain results from irritation or inflammation of pain-sensitive tissues within the functional unit. Improper static or inappropriate kinetic function can cause a painful reaction.

The appreciation of normal function is necessary before a true evaluation and interpretation can be made of the dysfunction in the causation of low back pain.

CHAPTER 2

Abnormal Deviation of Spinal Function As a Pain Factor

To know the normal and to recognize the deviation from normal; to be able to reproduce the pain by reproducing the abnormal position or movement; and to understand the mechanism by which the pain is caused—this is the formula for the clinical evaluation of the patient with low back pain.

The spine functioning in a proper static and kinetic manner should not elicit pain. The presence of pain indicates irritation of a pain-sensitive tissue at some point in the functional unit or in its adjacent tissues. Irritation of these tissues implies dysfunction of the spine, either from the *static* or the *kinetic* aspect.

LUMBOSACRAL ANGLE—STATIC SPINE

In the static spine the vast majority of painful states can be attributed to an increase in the lumbosacral angle with a consequent accentuation of the lumbar lordosis. This increase in the lumbar lordosis is commonly termed "sway back." It is a safe assumption to credit 75 per cent of all static or postural low back pains to such lordosis.

The lumbosacral angle is formed when the horizontal base of the angle is parallel to the ground level and the hypotenuse of the angle is formed at the level of the superior border of the sacrum (Fig. 17). The plane of the sacrum forms the base from which the lumbar spine takes off in its ascent and by which it achieves its balanced state.

The fifth lumbar vertebra lies upon the sacrum as a box rests on an inclined plane. The friction of the box on the incline, dependent on the weight of the box, prevents sliding, but there is the possibility of a sliding action down the incline plane which may constitute a shearing stress. As the angle of the sacrum increases, so does the slant of the inclined plane; thus the greater is the shearing stress (Fig. 18). Mathematically, an angle of 30 degrees will find the shearing stress to be 50 per cent of the superincumbent weight. An increase in the angle to 40 degrees will increase the shearing stress to 65 per cent of the superincumbent weight. Fifty degrees causes a shearing stress of approximately 75 per cent of the weight of the movable object.

Increase of the sacral angle not only increases the degree of shearing stress at the lumbosacral joint but by changing the angle of the base influences the curvature of the lordotic curve. The greater the angle of the take-off base the greater is the curve of the superincumbent spine insofar as the lumbar curve

33

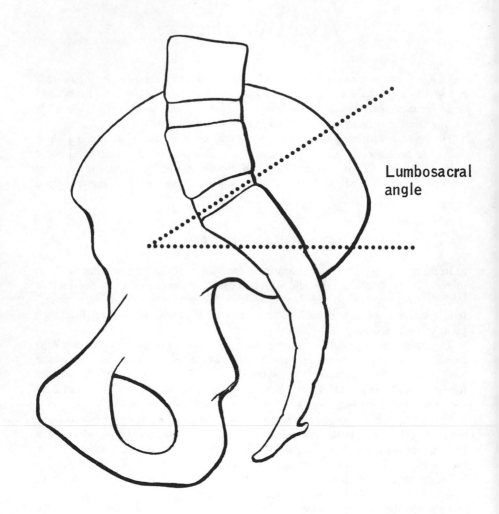

Lumbosacral
angle

FIGURE 17. Physiologic lumbosacral angle. The lumbosacral angle (LSA) is computed as the angle from a base parallel to horizontal and the hypotenuse drawn parallel to superior level of the sacral bone. The optimum physiologic lumbosacral is in the vicinity of 30 degrees.

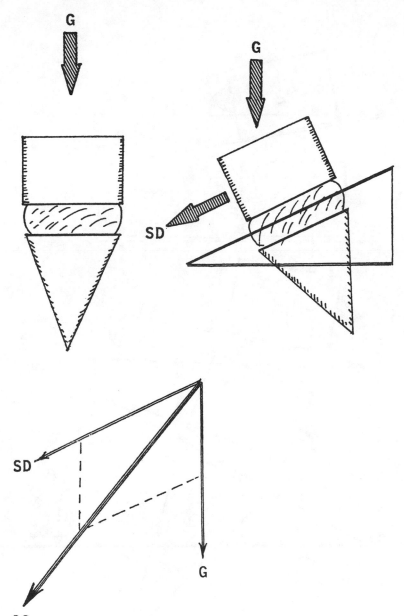

FIGURE 18.   Static shearing stress of the last lumbar vertebra in its inclined plane
relationship to the sacral vertebra.

G implies the gravity stress of the entire body upon the weight-bearing hydraulic
system of the intervertebral disk.

SD is the force of a body sliding down an inclined plane.

SS represents the resultant force and its direction of G and SD and is the shearing
stress exerted on the elastic fibers of the annulus.

35

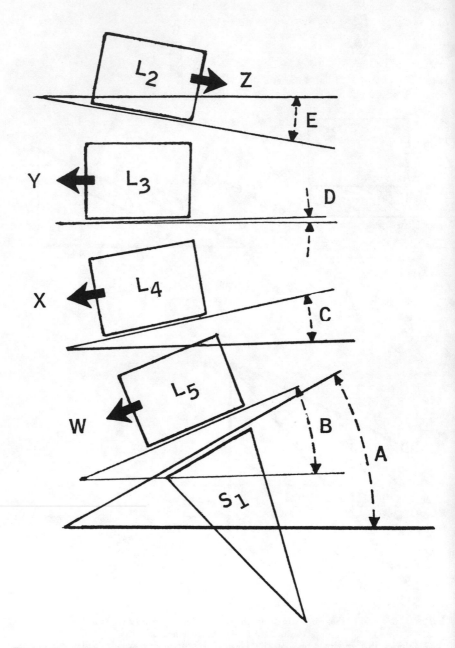

FIGURE 19. Differential shearing stress of lumbar vertebrae. The shearing stress of the last lumbar vertebra upon the first sacral differs from the shearing stresses of each successive cephalad vertebra. At each intervertebral level the inclined plane angle decreases and thus the shearing stress and its direction decreases (see text).

(lordosis) must always return to the plumb-line center and must do so within five vertebral segments. A more acute angle of the sacral base forms a less sharply curved lumbar spine because the lumber spine is then in more vertical position.

The degree of sacral angle influences the degree of angle of the fifth lumbar vertebra as computed to the horizontal base line. The shearing stress is proportional to the angle of the sacral inclination. The degree of angulation of the fourth vertebra on the fifth, the third on the fourth, the second on the third, decreases as the angle immediately below is decreased. The shearing stress correspondingly decreases proportionately with each successive ascending vertebral segment as the angle of inclination approaches the horizontal (Fig. 19). At the third lumbar vertebra the inclined plane, upon which it rests, is formed by the superior margin of the fourth lumbar vertebra and is almost horizontal; consequently there is only minimal tendency for the superimposed vertebra to slide forward and no shearing stress exists.

The anterior longitudinal ligament limits the extension of the lumbar spine. By its anterior attachment the opening of the intervertebral spaces is restricted. Any further attempt at extending the spine in this area results in closure of the posterior disk space (Fig. 20). Approximation of the posterior aspects of the vertebral bodies simultaneously approximate the posterior articulations.

When approximation of the posterior articulations causes a gliding of the facets into each other, they become weight-bearing units. Weight-bearing is not

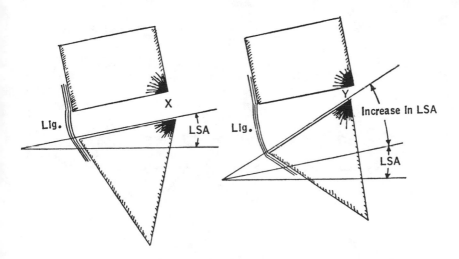

FIGURE 20. Mechanical analysis of posterior closure of the disk space by increase of the lumbosacral angle (LSA), anterior restriction of the anterior longitudinal ligament (Lig.). Narrowing of space X to space Y also portends approximation of the facets in their posterior relationship of the functional unit.

a physiologic function. When this occurs, the joint surfaces are compressed and synovial inflammation may result. Synovial inflammation is a pain-producing situation.

Besides the increase in lordosis that results from increase in sacral angulation, the increase in the incline causes greater shearing stress and places the facets in a position of "braking" action on the gliding superimposed vertebrae. This braking effort further compresses the articular synovial linings.

The so-called "sway back" posture is one of relaxation in which the person

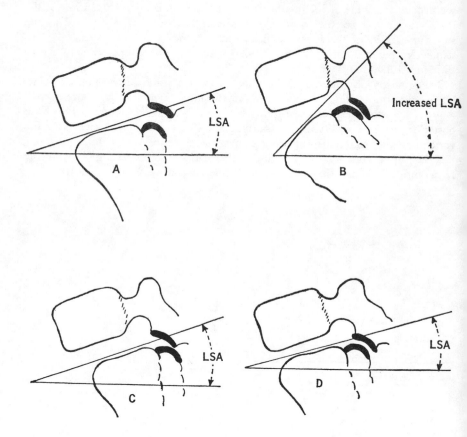

FIGURE 21. Variations in posterior articular relationships.

A, Normal lumbosacral angle with intact disk: normal relationship of articular facets.

B, Increase in lumbosacral angle (LSA) with posterior closure of the facets.

C, Spondylolisthesis with a normal LSA exerting traction on the posterior longitudinal ligament and disruption of facet alignment.

D, Disk degeneration with narrowing of intervertebral space and approximation of facets.

leans forward on his "Y" ligament while the pelvis shifts anterior to the center of gravity. The front portion of the pelvis cannot rotate upwards because of the restriction of the "Y" ligament; thus the sacral angle increases. The lumbar spine must curve back towards the center of gravity and does so by increasing its curvature. Thus the posture of "relaxation" is also a stance of ligamentous strain.

The first steps of the infant are characterized by marked lumbar lordosis. This posture is in part due to the failure of the iliopsoas muscles to elongate as the hips extend which failure places traction on the lumbar spine. It is also accentuated by weak hip-extensor and weak abdominal muscles. These latter factors play a part in the posture of the elderly or of the middle aged who are not in condition and whose posture may be described as slovenly.

The painful low back of pregnancy is related to an increase in lordosis. The gravid uterus causes a slight shift forward of the pelvis as it does also in the relaxed pose. Besides, there is a fatigue during pregnancy that deters good habits and efforts in addition to a hormonal ligamentous laxity that completes the picture.

The condition of "kissing spines" is described in which the posterior superior spines actually contact as the result of increased lordosis and its concomitant posterior joint approximation. The contact of the posterior spines and accompanying irritation cause a pseudoarthrosis to form. This condition, known as the syndrome of Baastrup, which occurs in patients under 25 years of age, finds the pain reduplicated by hyperextension of the spine. A pseudoarthrosis can be observed on x-ray.

Increase in the sacral angle will initiate or intensify the pain of spondylolysis and spondylolisthesis, a full consideration of which is given in Chapter 5. Various mechanisms of posterior articular derangement are pictured in Figure 21.

Pain which derives from increased lordosis because of approximation of the posterior segment in the functional unit has been attributed in part to facet impingement and irritation. Posterior articular approachment may also cause pain by irritating the nerve root as it emerges through the intervertebral foramen.

Hyperextension of the vertebral segment can mechanically irritate the nerve root (Fig. 22) and cause pain by compression of the main nerve or the branch of the recurrent nerve. This reaction can occur in the presence of a normal disk but with much greater facility when the increased angulation is combined with a narrowed disk space.

The majority of low back pain attributed to posture is related to increase in pelvic tilt, increase in lumbosacral angle, concomitant increase in lumbar lordosis, and the pain originating from irritation of the facet synovial tissue. Contact and friction of the posterior superior spines causing low back pain must also be part of the evaluation, but this is relatively a rare condition. Irritation of the nerve root at its site of foramen emergence is possible, but in this condition the resultant pain more likely would manifest itself in the dermatome distribution rather than as a pain exclusively located in the low back region. Irritation of the recurrent nerve and the synchronous muscle spasm will refer pain to the low back area.

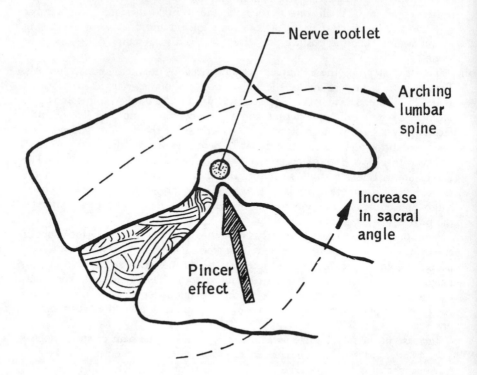

Nerve rootlet

Arching
lumbar
spine

Increase
in sacral
angle

Pincer
effect

FIGURE 22. Nerve root impingement due to hyperextension of the lumbosacral spine. Greater extent of impingement can be expected with a degenerated disk.

KINETIC LOW BACK PAIN

Pain caused by movement of the lumbar spine implies either a defective spine with impaired mechanical kinetics or a structurally normal spine functioning improperly. Kinetic pain implies irritation of pain-sensitive tissues activated by movements of the spine.

Pain may originate in the area of spine in one of *three* basic manners: (1) Abnormal strain on a normal back; (2) Normal stress on an abnormal back; (3) Normal stress on a normal back unprepared for the stress. The word *normal* as applied to strain implies a stress of reasonable magnitude that can be handled under average conditions without discomfort. A "normal" back refers to a structurally sound and functionally apt lumbar spine. The term *normal*, as always, has a relative value.

40

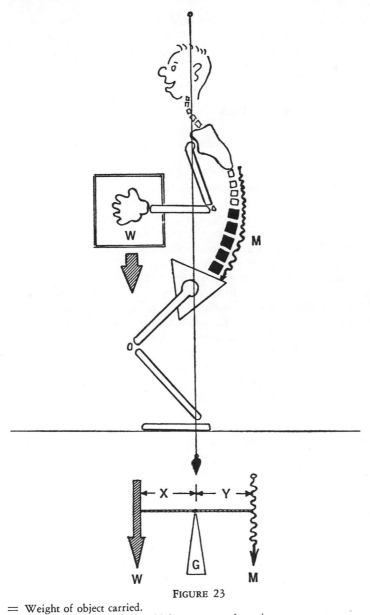

FIGURE 23

W   = Weight of object carried.
X   = Distance weight (W) is held from center of gravity.
Y   = Distance of spinal musculature from center of gravity.
M   = Tension developed by musculature.

$$W \times X = M \times Y$$

In a simple lever system the weight supported by the fulcrum (G) is the sum of the weights acting at each end of the lever bar.

100 x 10″ = 100 x 10″	G = 200 lbs.
100 x 20″ = 200 x 10″	G = 300 lbs.

A good example of abnormal stress would be that of a person who suddenly has to catch a falling weight of several hundred pounds. Such an act would constitute an excessive stress that would overwhelm the muscles and ligaments of a normal back.

Abnormal Strain on Normal Back

A normal back, by the combination of muscle ˙contraction which reduces the strain of the ligamentous structure can sustain a superimposed weight for a reasonable period of time. If the object which a person must hold immediately before him is too heavy, muscular contraction may be insufficient. As the object is held farther away from the body, muscular tone decreases because the value of the fulcrum decreases (Fig. 23). Holding even a reasonable weight at a reasonable distance from the body for too long a period of time will cause muscular fatigue or exhaustion (Fig. 24).

When muscular contraction has been overcome or exhausted the brunt of the stress falls on the ligaments which have a limited resiliency and once the ligaments give way the stress falls on the joints and subluxation of the joint results. Pain can manifest itself many times during this sequence of events. Sustained muscular contraction can produce ischemia in the muscle tissue, capable of causing pain. Excessive strain on the myofascial attachment to the periosteum may also result in pain. Painful capsular stretch may follow the loss of the ligamentous "protection" that normally guards the joints.

Any overwhelming stress will stretch the ligaments of the functional unit, exceed the movement within the unit and ultimately stretch the long ligaments throughout the entire spine. Not only segmental instability may result but it is possible that the physiologic curves of the spine may be altered. As previously stated, overwhelming stress may be caused by an extraordinary weight imposed on the supporting structure, by an average weight held in a markedly eccentric manner, or by a light object held for unduly long periods of time.

Normal Strain on Abnormal Back

Normal use of an abnormal back implies proper utilization of a structurally defective back. Sometimes due to a defect in the spine or its contiguous tissues, the stress may be improper or excessive. This defect may be found in the bony structures, the articular portions of the spine, the ligaments, the muscular tissues, or in any of these combinations.

In a *structural scoliosis* the facets are not parallel in a symmetrical plane because of the lateral curving and associated rotation of the vertebral segments. Bending and extending in an anterior posterior direction that occur normally at the lumbar segment must now be done with the facets in an oblique position. The gliding movement is attempted by the asymmetrical facets, and smooth movement of one pair of facets upon the other is impaired, with a loss of facile action and the limitation of total movement. When movement is forced past

42

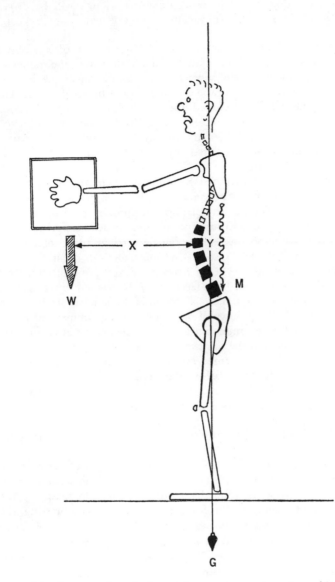

FIGURE 24. Increase of strain imposed upon erect spine when object of same weight is held at arm's length.

W = 100 lbs.	W x X = M x Y
X = 24″	100 x 24 = M x 6
Y = 6″	M = 400 lbs.

M + W = 500 lbs. (G)

By increasing any component of a simple lever arm the total weight superimposed on the supporting structure can be altered. Either changing the weight of the held object or increasing the distance from the body will increase the gravity (G) strain and will concurrently increase the muscular stress (M) as the distance Y changes little if any. The M stress is a muscular compressive force on the vertebral disks.

the point that the facet alignment will now permit, the joints will be driven together and impacted. This is rightfully called "impingement" or "freezing" of the facets.

Two different mechanics may cause pain in the movement of a scoliotic spine. Rotation of a segment of the spinal column decreases the range of normal physiologic movement of that segment. This limitation occurs because the facets now assume a position at an angle to their usual plane of action. The ligaments along the spine follow this curved line and thus shorten. Spinal flexion past a certain degree is met by mechanical structural restriction, and any exertion of force will result in overstretch of the tissues. In this type of movement restriction the pain mechanism initiated by forced flexion occurs from ligamentous-articular-capsular stretch.

The second pain mechanism attributed to scoliosis occurs as the spine re-extends from the flexed position. As the spine extends and approaches the erect lumbar lordotic curve, the posterior articulations reapproximate. Parallel symmetrical facets with smooth synovial lining permit unimpeded reapproachment. The presence of facet asymmetry causes the female carriage to be oblique to the entering male portion of the facets, so that impingement can result.

The impingement of facets as they arise from the flexed position which occurs from structural asymmetry of the facets may be caused by a similar mechanism when the spine has a *functional* scoliosis. Functional scoliosis can occur from a unilateral limited hip range of motion impeding symmetrical pelvic rotation. Impingement is further augmented when a person resumes an erect position after flexion and violates the lumbar-pelvic rhythm in reverse. This infraction of the rhythm can best be termed *two-stage* extension of the spine because the lumbar lordosis is resumed before the pelvic derotation has reached its *proportionate* relationship of the lumbosacral rhythm. *Two-stage* re-extension may cause impingement of the facets even in the absence of scoliosis if the reascent is done rapidly, with force, and if the body is contorted during the action (Fig. 25). In this case the rotated spine position causes functional facet asymmetry.

The site from which pain emanates in this impingement mechanism is the articular synovial tissue. The facets impinge and compress the adjacent synovial tissues causing an acute synovitis. Immediate protective muscle spasm of the segment follows with the compressive force of the spasm compressing the interposed disk and simultaneously causing further impaction of the posterior facets. Clinically this syndrome is called an *acute facet impingement.*

Normal use of an abnormal back resulting in pain occurs also when *tight hamstrings* are present. The lumbar spine is not abnormal, but the lumbar-pelvic rhythm has a malfunctioning cog in its mechanism. Full painless movement of the spine requires complete rotation of the pelvis as well as total reversal of the lumbar lordotic curve. Inflexible hamstring muscles by their attachment from the posterior knee region to the ischial tuberosity of the pelvis prevent full rotation. In total body flexion, once the pelvis has reached its maximum rotation, if total flexion has not been reached, further bending may be forced by more lumbar curving. As further bending of the lumbar spine is prevented by the posterior longitudinal ligaments, insistence will result in

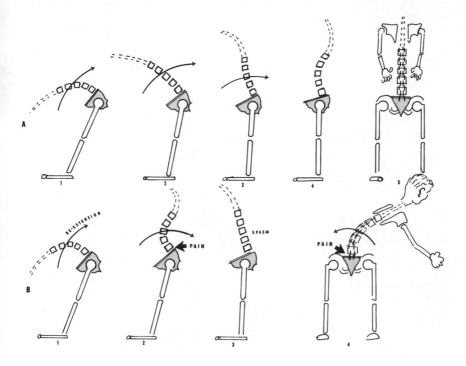

FIGURE 25. Mechanism of acute facet impingement. A, 1 through 5 depict the proper physiologic resumption of the erect position from total flexion with reverse *lumbar-pelvic* rhythm. Re-extension must be in the anterior posterior plane as shown in A, 5. B shows improper premature return of lordotic curve before adequate pelvic de-rotation (B, 2). This cantilevers the lumbar spine anterior to the center of gravity and approximates the facets causing *pain* (B, 2). With the body flexed and rotated there is further asymmetry of the facets facilitating unilateral impingement (B, 4).

ligamentous stretch pain. Tearing of the ligamentous-periosteal fibrous attachment may actually result, if not a tear in the ligament itself. Repeated overstretching leads to instability of that segment owing to the elongation of the restrictive ligaments (Fig. 26).

The "tight low back" produces pain in a manner converse to that of the tight restrictive hamstrings. In the tight low back mechanism the pelvic rotation phase of the lumbar-pelvic rhythm is free and full, but the lumbar-flexion phase is impeded. Instead of the lumbar lordosis physiologically flexing synchronously with the rotation of the pelvic area, the pelvis rotates and the lumbar curve, having gone as far as the tight paraspinous tissues will permit, ceases. At this point the low back attempts to flex further but cannot. Further forcing will cause painful stretching of the posterior longitudinal ligament, the capsule of the articulations, and the fibrous elements of the paraspinous muscles.

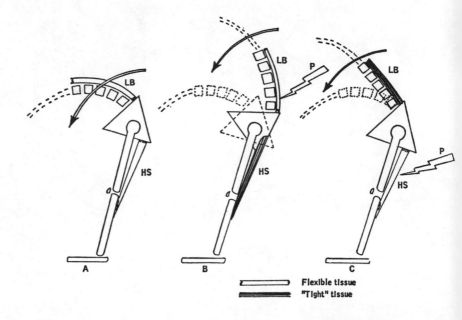

FIGURE 26. Mechanism of stretch pain in the "tight hamstring" and the "tight low back" syndromes. A, Normal flexibility with unrestricted lumbar-pelvic rhythm. B, Tight hamstrings (HS) restricting pelvic rotation and thereby causing excessive stretch of low back (LB) resulting in pain (P). C, Tight low back (LB) performing an incomplete lumbar reversal and thus, by placing excessive stretch on the hamstrings (HS), causes pain (P) in both the hamstrings and the low back as well as a disrupted lumbar-pelvic rhythm.

Normal Stress on an Unprepared Normal Back

The third concept of body mechanics dysfunction that may result in low back pain is the concept of normal stress imposed on a normal back but imposed at a moment when the back is unprepared for such stress.

Any musculoskeletal physical activity is preceded by anticipation and preparation. Muscular contraction is needed to initiate movement. The anticipated movement is graded to the required intensity of contraction, to the rapidity of contemplated action, and to the extent of contraction necessary for time and space factors. Contemplation of the ultimate action computes all these factors, and the contraction is then initiated. Too much contraction will "overshoot the mark" and cause excessive movement at the articulation upon which the muscular action is directed. Too much movement of the joint can cause movement in a faulty direction or can exceed the normal physiologic range of that joint motion. Damage to the joint and periarticular tissues is apt to result.

Under the proper conditions an impending stress in which a counteraction is anticipated will cause the body to react with just the right tone and contraction to receive the stress. Too little tone will allow the stress to overcome the muscular action, and the stress will bear its full impact on the ligaments. Too much tone or excessive muscular countercontraction will cause a rebound in the opposite direction to the stress and thus again subject the joint or joints to undue strain.

The appropriate use of the term *normal* in its relation to stress may be questioned. Can stress be considered normal if the end result of the stress causes damage or irritation to tissues, which are in themselves normal. By *normal* must be understood that which would be a tolerable stress under ordinary conditions. Lifting a suitcase thought to be empty when it is really heavily loaded will cause the back to use a weak contraction rather than the necessary adequate setting and contraction. Strain can result although the loaded suitcase can be lifted without strain or discomfort when the individual is prepared. The object causing stress is certainly of normal weight but it catches the back unprepared. The evolution of the anticipated contraction was inept.

Similar to the faulty setting of the anticipated "grading for the job," as in the example just given, is the case of a person whose personality, emotional state, or degree of impatience at the time of the action results in improper calibration of the resulting muscular contraction. The tense person acting in an abrupt, taut manner will usually perform muscular feats with an inaccurate gradient of effort and in a mechanically erratic manner.

More than the necessary muscle strength will be used by the person who is impatient to have the job finished or who is distracted and inattentive to the demands of the task. These people bend quickly to finish what they have to do before their muscles are set. Such people arise abruptly from a flexed position in the "two-stage" manner rather than by smooth reversal of the lumbar-pelvic rhythm. Frequently in a state of anxiety or tension proper learned patterns are easily forgotten.

Electromyographic studies have confirmed the inefficiency of muscular effort in nervous tense people. In the performance of a simple motor task normally requiring a relatively few motor units acting toward one end, people who are tense, nervous, or anxious, display simultaneous and marked discharge of motor units throughout the entire body. Muscles totally unrelated and unneeded react in varying states of contractility. Not only does this excessive motor activity cause inefficiency of energy expenditure, but because of non-integrated contraction of muscles smooth motor activity cannot possibly result.

A person with a normal back that is muscularly fatigued from prolonged activity and subjected to a stress considered normal may respond with a muscular reaction that is inadequate in strength, endurance, or timing. Can a "fatigued" back be considered normal? If the back is not found to be abnormal, it is unprepared then for the task presented.

47

Each repeated condition that results in back pain undoubtedly leaves its tell-tale mark on the back until the degree of normalcy of the back decreases and a previously tolerable stress now becomes an abnormal one.

SUMMARY

Low back pain results from deviation of normal posture in the *static spine* and from deviation of normal function in the *kinetic spine*. Irritation of pain-sensitive tissues must occur before pain is elicited. Normal posture and normal kinetics in a normal spine do not initiate pain.

Low back discomfort in the *static* spine occurs primarily from an increase in the lumbosacral angle which in turn increases the lumbar lordosis. Most cases of postural low back pain must be attributed to an accentuated "sway back."

Low back pain resulting during or from movement of the spine can be attributed to violation of the *lumbar-pelvic rhythm*. The *rhythmic* pattern may be faulty in its performance or some of the functional segments of the spine that participate in the rhythm may be inadequate.

Any consideration of low back pain must keep in mind the factors of abnormal stress on the normal spine, abnormal stress on a mechanically normal spine, and the imposition of a usually normal stress on a mechanically normal spine but imposed at a time when the back is not ready to receive the stress.

It is now possible to turn to the patient who suffers from backache and apply to clinical use the knowledge of functional anatomy and the recognition of possible painful deviations.

CHAPTER 3

Clinical Application of Low Back Mechanics in the Diagnosis and Treatment of Pain Syndromes

The history and physical examination of the patient with low back pain must have as its objective a *functional* diagnosis based on static and kinetic appreciation of the patient's spine and its relation to the normal.

LOCALIZATION OF PAIN BY HISTORY TAKING

It may be trite to say that the patient's claim of "pain in the low back" is not necessarily an accurate statement. Localizing the pain in the lower back region is the problem since the patient may be vague and obscure.

Many a patient will often designate the wrong organ eliciting his pain like the patient with a pain in his "kidney area" when actually the pain exists in the lumbosacral area or the patient with a pain in his "hip" when the pain is really in the sacroiliac region. But the site of the pain can easily be localized if the patient is asked to point with his finger tips to the spot in pain. The site so specified has more anatomic localization than do the descriptive words of the patient.

A description of the characteristic of the pain is valuable. Words by the patient, such as "dull," "sharp," or "burning," have significance in that certain tissues when irritated will cause pain of that specified type and description. The site of the tissues (responsible for this type of pain) in the functional unit or along the entire spine has obvious localizing value.

Frequency and duration of pain have both diagnostic and prognostic significance. Mechanical instability of the back can be suspected when there is frequent recurrence of painful attacks. The duration of pain varies also with the type and site of tissue irritated. This gives insight into the recuperative powers of the patient. The amount of disability claimed by the patient to result from the pain gives the experienced examiner his first insight into the pain-threshold of the patient. The pain-tolerance of a patient is difficult to evaluate accurately.

After the localization of the pain has been determined, the case history will next seek the *"when"* and *"how"* of the pain-producing mechanism. A description of the *when* in relation to time of day or to type of work or activity is presented when the patient states, "It happens only when . . . ." The *when* thus also becomes a *how* presenting some clarification of the mechanism of the pain production. The patient's description of the time and manner of *when* and *how* differentiates the pain in its *static* or *kinetic* nature.

PHYSICAL EXAMINATION

Examination is fundamentally an attempt to reproduce by deliberate actions and movements the patient's symptoms. A basic axiom follows: *If the characteristic pain can be produced by a position or by a movement, and the exact nature of that position and movement is completely understood, the mechanism of the pain production is understood.*

At precisely the position or the moment of the movement at which pain is produced, by knowing what is occurring in the body mechanics and by appreciating the deviation of this movement or position from normal function, the physician discovers the mechanism of pain production. As has been discussed, the history has already alluded to the general classification of static or kinetic and the patient himself has suggested the *where, when,* and *how* of his pain. The examination now confirms the clinical impression implied by the history.

General Observations

The physical examination has already begun as the history is being taken. The manner in which the patient enters the office, and his sitting or standing posture as the history is recorded are significantly revealing. The static posture has already been observed, and an insight into the patient's emotional tone as portrayed by his postural attitude has been gained. (Refer to Chapter 1, pp. 15-18.)

Likewise, the handshake, too often overlooked and too infrequently interpreted, is an exceeding valuable portion of any physical examination. The basic personality often is revealed in a person's handshake. The handshake is as revealing a depiction of the emotional tone as is posture.

The limp "dead fish" or "wet rag" handshake usually indicates a listless individual whose symptoms are in part influenced by this hypokinetic attitude and who can be expected to put very little effort into an energetic treatment program that the doctor will prescribe for him.

The "bone crushing" or "pump handle" handshake indicates a hyperkinetic compulsive type in spite of the impression he wishes to create.

In contrast is the firm reassuring handshake, when related to similiar postural appearance and the objective history that is being noted, which gives the examiner a feeling of security in the integrity of the story the patient tells and confidence that the patient will try to carry out the prescribed treatment.

The history must carefully evaluate previous therapeutic attempts, and the reason for past failures must be judged carefully. Failure to improve from a program that once was deemed to be correct either stimulates a need for further studies or questions the accuracy of the patient's history. One or the other is in error.

The possibility of inaccurate diagnosis must also be considered. Again, failure of patient cooperation may indicate lack of understanding on the part of the patient or poor instructions that had been given by the former therapist. Another possibility must always be kept in mind, namely, that a patient may psychologically need either consciously or subconsciously his symptoms and will relinquish them reluctantly. This evaluation must be made very cautiously, but the truth may be suspected when the patient implies a "happiness" over treatment failures, "everything has been tried," and "the best doctors have been puzzled," etc. The "pleasure from failure" is paradoxical but real.

The physical examination of the patient is best performed in a progressive-systematized pattern. This routine need not be stereotyped or inflexible, but the examination should be performed in an orderly sequence that tends to preclude omission of essential details.

The patient should be sufficiently undressed to permit adequate observation of the static and kinetic aspects of the body. The male patient can undress to his undershorts. The female patient must be exposed but must have protection against encroachment upon modesty. A gown of knee-length which is open in the back but adequately fastened to permit movement should suffice for the examination.

Evaluation of Posture (Static Spine)

The patient's posture has had a cursory examination when he enters the examining room and during the history portion of the interview. In the examining room the patient is intentionally and obviously examined for posture. He or she is aware of the scrutiny. This pose may be revealing. A pose may be assumed portraying what is considered to be proper posture, or it may be the pose that depicts the painful state or the feelings he wishes to portray. This projection of posture may be either unconscious or intentional, and the motivation is not always easily discerned. The posture assumed by the patient is always revealing, but the revelation assumes importance only insofar as it is correctly interpreted and properly used in diagnosis.

The examiner begins by observing the patient from a side view, with especial concentration on the lumbar curvature, the opposite curve of the dorsal spine, and the relative position of the hips, knees, and feet in relation to an assumed plumb line of gravity. The cervical spine, although not to be stressed here, cannot fail to be considered in the total aspect of body posture. This cervical curve must conform to the other curves and is a significant determinant of posture.

51

Pelvic Level—Leg Length

Posterior viewing of the static spine should first take into consideration the level of the pelvis. Determining the pelvic level is essentially an evaluation of leg length. To measure the length of each leg by tape measure from malleolus to anterior-superior spine or iliac crest is at best inaccurate and offers little practical significance. Ascertaining comparative leg lengths is of greatest value insofar as the legs through their upright supporting structure influence the level of the pelvis. This horizontal pelvic plane is the foundation of the spinal take-off, and its level can only be determined by examining the patient in the upright position.

The patient is examined standing barefooted with both legs close together and both legs fully extended at the knees. The pelvic level is then determined in three manners. The examiner places the fingertips of his hands upon the pelvic brim on each side. By sitting back, at arms' length, the examiner can determine the horizontal level of his fingertips and hence the level of the iliac crests. The accuracy of this measure is surprisingly precise and the differences of as little as one quarter of an inch can be estimated.

The "dimples" noted in most people in the region of the sacroiliac joints can be "lined up" by the eye and furnish another estimate of pelvic level. These dimples are located parasacrally where the gluteus maximus muscle attaches to the periosteum overlying the sacrum. Except in very obese or in very thin people, these dimples can easily be observed.

Observation of the lumbar spine in its take-off or in the angle of ascent from the sacrum presents a third method of determining pelvic level. The posterior-superior spines of the vertebrae are usually prominent and can be seen along the floor of the valley created by the erector-spinae muscle masses. The lumbar spine ordinarily takes off from the sacral base at right angles in a straight vertical direction. If an oblique take-off is noted, it indicates that the spine is curved or implies obliquity of the sacral base. These three methods of measuring leg length are used to determine the level of the pelvis only insofar as it influences lumbar spine take-off from its sacral base. The conclusion drawn from the three methods is significantly accurate.

If these three clinical methods of determining pelvic obliquity indicate any leg length discrepancy, the exact degree of leg length difference can be determined. Boards of known thickness can be placed under the foot of the short leg until the pelvis reaches the level determined by the above three methods. The thickness of the board establishes the degree of leg length difference. The boards of varying thicknesses of ⅛, ¼, ½, ¾, and 1 inch can be used in various combinations until the pelvic level has reached the horizontal. It must be remembered that a straight vertical spine rather than a level pelvis is desired. Achieving a level pelvis is merely a means towards this end.

When a significant leg length discrepancy exists, the cause of the difference will usually be revealed by further observations and appropriate studies. Unilateral *genu valgum* or *genu varum* may be a sufficient degree to cause a change in total leg length. Atrophy of a leg due to posterior poliomyelitis or to previous fracture or surgical intervention is easily discernible. Regardless of the cause, the significance of leg length shortening resides in its effect on the pelvic level and ultimately in its effect on the spinal alignment.

At this stage in the examination the static spine, posture is evident. The physiologic curves with their relationship to pelvic angulation have been ascertained, and the erectness of the spine from a posterior view has been sufficiently verified to assume proper facet alignment. The major factors influencing the static posture have been established so that it is possible now to consider the kinetics of the spine.

Lumbar-Pelvic Rhythm

Asking the patient to "bend forward in an attempt to touch your toes" but requesting that this flexion be done "without bending the knees" initiates the first phase of the lumbar-pelvic rhythm. These two requests have intentionally been placed within quotation marks. Observation of the bending forward "with knees stiff" permits evaluation of the freedom permitted rotation at the hip joints. Hamstring tightness is also revealed by this specific request. The stiff knees also insure maintenance of the horizontal pelvic level as ascertained from the posterior view of the static spine while leg length was being measured. A short leg that influences the static stance also must influence the kinetic spine by altering the vertical alignment of the spine. Bending one knee will cause that leg to be temporarily shorter than the fully extended leg.

"Bend *as if* to try to touch your toes" is requested of the patient because the ability to touch one's toes is not had by all and in no sense of the word implies normalcy. To infer that such flexibility is expected of the patient is fallacious insofar as a large percentage of people, regardless of their age, cannot, never have, and probably never will be able to touch their toes, and yet are functionally adequate and flex in a pain-free manner. The main reason for asking the patient to perform this feat is to observe the *manner* of bending rather than to *measure* the *extent* of total flexion.

As the patient bends forward, the smoothness of the lumbar-curve reversal is observed. The ratio of this reversal is noted in respect to the pelvic rotation. The correlation of the two simultaneous movements is observed. In essence the lumbar-pelvic rhythm is studied. Each component of the movement is observed, and the relationship to each other in the rhythm is ascertained. Failure of the lumbar lordosis to reverse during flexion may indicate protective muscle spasm or mechanical restriction because of malfunction of the joints, capsules, ligaments, or muscles of the lumbar spine. Interruption of the pelvic rotation limiting the total lumbar-pelvic movement may imply tight hamstring muscles, irritable sciatic nerve, or inability of the pelvis to rotate on its hip-joint axis owing to faulty hip joints.

The simultaneous lumbar-flexion action with the concomitant pelvic rotation should be a smooth action with each aspect being reasonably complete. Restriction of either portion of the action indicates the phase of the rhythm that is defective.

If pain is elicited during the performance of this "bending forward" test, the observer must be immediately informed of the exact moment "when" the pain is felt and "where" it is felt. The "when" refers to the moment during the lumbar-pelvic flexion rotation at which the existence of pain is noticed and the "where" indicates the area of the back (or leg) at which the patient localizes the pain. Evaluation of the discrepancy in the rhythm, and the existence of pain at the moment when the discrepancy is noted reveals the mechanism of the pain. The "where" may denote a general area but when combined with a description of the pain intimates a more specific tissue site.

The patient himself indicates the "when" of the pain at the time the pain occurs during the bending exercise. This process fulfills the axiom "when I can reproduce pain and at the same time know what is happening, at that very moment I understand the mechanism of the pain."

Limited pelvic rotation around the transverse axis of the hip joints is frequently caused by "tight" hamstrings. Tight hamstrings signify inability of the muscles of the hamstring group to elongate because of excessive intramuscular connective tissue of limited elasticity. Usually the hamstrings which are inelastic bilaterally and symmetrically restrict pelvis rotation. Unilateral hamstring limitation will cause asymmetrical pelvic limitation in addition to a rotatory trunk flexion. Ultimate testing in straight leg raising range will reveal the extent of hamstring elasticity. Sciatic nerve-stretch pain also produces unilateral restriction of pelvic rotation and interferes with the smooth lumbar-pelvic rhythm.

The observation of the pathway traversed by the entire spine during its total flexion may reveal a functional scoliosis that in the static erect position was not apparent. Facet asymmetry may be revealed during flexion by its effect on the course and direction of the spinal flexion. Scoliosis may result, it must be remembered, by a pelvic obliquity caused by a short leg and this scoliosis may become more apparent during spine flexion even though it exists also in the erect posture.

Having observed the patient flex fully and slowly, and having observed the fulfillment of the flexion phase of the lumbar-pelvic rhythm, the physician will now ask the patient to return slowly to the erect position. After reaching the fully bent over position, he must be warned that the reverse flexion be performed slowly.

Reversed lumbar-pelvic rhythm in extension is now to be observed. The gradual return of the lumbar flexion to the erect position of lordosis with smooth simultaneous reverse rotation of the pelvis to its physiologic sacral angle should be the exact reversal of the rhythm observed during flexion. During re-extension, the pelvis should gradually resume its position over the plumb-line center of gravity. Proper "uncurling" should be smooth, symmetrical, and painless.

Should pain or discomfort be noted during re-extension, the exact moment and the exact point of the extension mechanism should be noted. At the instant in the re-extension cycle when pain is evoked a discrepancy in the lumbar-pelvic rhythm can usually be observed. The most frequent divergence in the rhythm is that of a premature return of the lumbar spine lordosis with the reverse rotation of the pelvis lagging. The lumbar lordosis is resumed before the pelvis establishes itself beneath the lumbar curve and is adequately de-rotated. At this stage of re-extension the lumbar spine should be in its erect lordotic phase and the sacral base should have returned to its proper erect supporting angle, but we find the pelvis is still tilted and thus the take-off of the lumbar spine occurs in a forward slant. The lumbar spine is cantilevered anteriorly to the center of gravity.

Because of the premature lumbar lordosis the spine is eccentrically loaded, and muscular action is needed to maintain it in this off-center balance. This position is inefficient and fatiguing. In its attempt to achieve balance over the proper center of gravity the lumbar spine will arc, that is, increase its lordosis and thus further approximate the posterior articulations. The combined "arching backwards" and the added muscular contraction to maintain the eccentric balance further compress the facets' together and cause them to become weight-bearing. Diagrammatically, the reverse of flexion is depicted in Fig. 14 viewed in reverse, and the faulty mechanism of de-rotation is shown in Fig. 27.

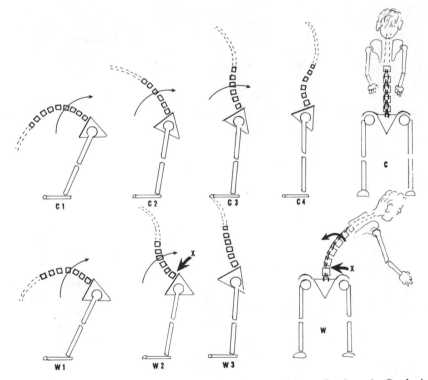

FIGURE 27. Faulty re-extension from the bent-over position. C_1 through C_4 depict gradual re-extension by simultaneously rotating the pelvis as the lumbar spine moves from reversed lordosis into erect lumbar lordosis. With the spine straight, as in C, the facets move properly. W_1 through W_3 depict improper re-extension where at W_3 the lumbar spine has become already "arched" before the pelvis has adequately rotated in a proper *lumbar-pelvic rhythm*. If the person is also rotated during this re-extension motion, his facets can "jam" during return to erect position and the disks are subjected to additional stress from the torque motion.

55

The kinetic examination proceeds with the patient continuing to arch further backwards. This extension after the patient has reached his static posture is, therefore, a position of hyperextension. This maneuver further increases the lumbar lordosis, the posterior articulations are more approximated, the center of gravity moves backwards, and the pelvis must, therefore, shift forward to keep the patient in balance. A marked "sway back" is created by this position. If pain results, similar to that previously complained of by the patient, the mechanism of the pain is revealed. Increase of the lumbar lordosis with posterior articular approximation is the cause. It must be admitted that this extreme "arching backwards" cannot be considered a daily ritual or an everyday occurrence, but the mechanism of pain production is basic. The graphic "arching" due to hyperextension is depicted in Fig. 26C, and the pelvic relationship to the center of gravity is clearly apparent.

So far in the examination the *static* or postural and *kinetic* or functional spine have been evaluated both from the lateral view and the anterior-posterior aspect. We may possibly have reduplicated the patient's pain and thereby have revealed the mechanism of pain production. The severity of the pain may not have been reduplicated as the production of severe pain demands more factors than the circumstances of the examination permit. What is significant is the reproduction of the pain by a controlled position or action.

Additional clinical tests that augment and confirm the diagnostic picture must include an adequate neurologic evaluation. This will be discussed in some detail in the chapter on disk disease.

SUMMARY

The patient who presents himself with a complaint of low-back pain is evaluated by means of the case history and by specific physical examination. The history indicates *where, when,* and *how* the pain occurs. The *static* or the *kinetic* nature of the dysfunction is specified.

The *where* of the pain given in the history furnishes an anatomic localization; the *when* implies the time of movement, the nature of the movement, and the relationship to environmental factors that may be relevant. The *how* of the pain is divulged to the examiner who is cognizant of different mechanisms which may possibly cause pain. The characteristics of the pain described corroborates in part the suspected tissues involved as indicated in the history.

The examination, by permitting observation of *static* structure and the performance of *kinetic* function, leads to a functional diagnosis. If the normal is known regarding *static* and *kinetic* spinal function and appearance, the deviation from this normal can be appraised.

The axiom now applies: *"If characteristic pain can be reproduced by a position or by a movement and the exact nature of that position and movement is fully comprehended, the mechanism of the pain is understood."*

The treatment which follows must change, where possible, the static posture and correct the faulty kinetics. The tissues that make these corrections possible must be strengthened where necessary, made more flexible when deemed essential, and the neuromuscular patterns must be established and repeated until the operation is easy, automatic, and constant in its performance.

CHAPTER 4

Correction of Faulty Mechanics in Therapeutic Approach to Low Back Pain

After evaluation of the normal mechanism of back function, both from a static viewpoint and a kinetic status, treatment must essentially be a correction of what has been found to be faulty. A position or a movement which is contrary to normal movement and normal position and which reduplicates the pain complaint must be corrected.

FAULTY POSTURE CONCEPTS

The treatment of faulty posture causing static pain is fundamentally simple in its prescription. Insofar as faulty and painful posture is usually one of increased lordosis the treatment is to teach a *flat low-back* exercise. The increase in lordosis is dependent on the lumbosacral angle; therefore, the remedy is to change the pelvic angle. In essence *"tuck in the pelvis"* is the instruction.

The concept of the *tuck in* may be difficult for the patient to understand or feel. Since sway-back posture usually has been of long duration, the pattern is now well established. Even though lordotic posture will be causative of pain, this increase in lumbar arch *is* the *natural*, effortless postural pattern and in the patient there is likely inherent tendency to resist change, especially when effort and repeated effort must be made.

The factors that led to the original formation of this postural pattern are well established and are not easily broken. The familial tendency in the patient may frequently lead to a pessimism that "the condition runs in my family and is beyond my control." Minimal effort resulting in no immediate results may be sufficiently discouraging to some patients to end all further efforts. What is considered maximum effort for some patients is minimal cooperation for others, and vice versa. The constitutional variants and the psychologic factors that enter into cooperation can frequently tax the doctor. Serious questions concerning the correctness of diagnosis and prescribed treatment may arise in the mind of the doctor when the patient states, "I have done the exercises faithfully for months, and my back still hurts in the same way when I stand."

Adherence by the patient to his prescribed exercise program must be constantly and frequently supervised and reviewed. When these same exercises are later demonstrated to the doctor by the patient, it is amazing how distorted prescribed exercises may become a few weeks after the initial description by the doctor. The method or manner of doing these exercises may have no resemblance to that prescribed. Again, the reason for doing the exercises may frequently not be understood and must time and again be retaught. The addition of other exercises that neutralize the value of the prescribed regime occasionally are added by the patient himself. These neutralizing exercises are usually of the back-arching, hyperextension variety. Such exercises will be discussed in more detail in the section on exercises.

Probably the greatest failure occurs in the case of the patient who does his exercises faithfully but fails to "carry over" the posture to everyday activities. The performance of exercises is basically a training device and must be integrated into every activity of everyday living. Posture is a full-time function of the body and must be maintained properly during every waking hour— standing, walking, sitting, in fact, in any upright stance. To exercise merely one hour a day every day and stand in a faulty manner the remainder of the 15 hours in which the patient is awake will lead to no improvement in posture and no decrease in pain.

For the patient whose posture is a portrayal of his emotional state there will obviously be little or no carry-over. In the chronically depressed person, more than exercise is needed. Drugs may help and even psychiatric intervention may be necessary. Such posture is the "picture" the patient wishes to portray to the world for his own psyche satisfaction; treatment from strictly mechanical-postural approach will fail.

Fatigue plays a large part in failure. In the psychasthenic person who does not possess a constitutional potential for endurance, no amount of exercise, drugs, or even corseting will give the necessary stamina, ligamentous tone, and muscle tone. The person does not have the resources, and as the muscle tone leaves the patient the ligaments become the only support and pain ensues.

There is the acceptable fatigue that occurs in everyone who reaches then exceeds his tolerance by hard work, prolonged activity, inadequate rest, or who is performing tasks for which he is anatomically or physically not suited. The problem in such instances is the recognition of these fatigue factors and the ability of the patient to make the necessary changes.

When the consideration of all these factors indicates that the problem is mechanical and demands flat-back treatment, pelvic-tilting exercises and their functional application must be taught and utilized.

PELVIC-TILTING EXERCISES

Initially, pelvic tilting is easier taught when the patient lies in a supine position. A firm surface upon which the patient lies supine is preferable to a soft surface, as it permits greater awareness of the points of body contact. After pelvic tilting has been mastered in a supine position, it must ultimately be performed in the upright position. The concept of this ultimate transition must be kept in mind from the onset.

The exercise is begun with the person lying supine in a comfortable position,

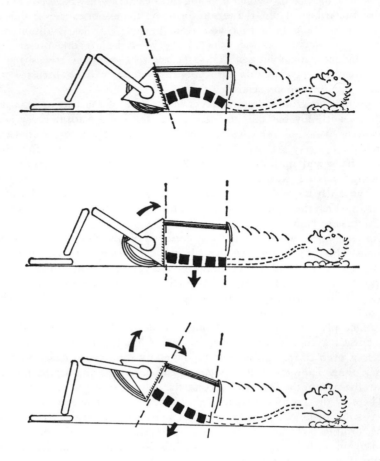

FIGURE 28. Pelvic-tilting exercises done in supine position. A, First step: supine position with hips and knees flexed. B, Second step: lumbar spine is pressed down to the floor. C, Third step: holding lumbar spine firmly to the floor the buttocks are elevated from the floor thus "tilting" the pelvis while keeping a "flat" back.

hips and knees flexed, both feet flat on the floor, and the head relaxed on a pillow. In this position the first movement is that of the patient forcing or "pressing" his lower back down flat to the floor. This movement is performed by the combined contraction of the abdominal and the gluteal muscles, but the effect is "felt" by the patient in his hamstring and quadriceps muscles as well. A "squeezing" sensation of the hips and thighs is experienced. Placing the patient's hand at the "small" of the back and having him press down on his hand may help him in understanding the intended movement. A sharp object may be used beneath the back to give the patient an awareness of the proper feeling of the posture.

A pillow under the patient's head will obviate any strain which may arise from stress in supporting the head or from improper breathing during the course of the exercise. Neck strain may become so distracting that it overshadows the concept of proper pelvic movement.

Once the lower back is pressing against the floor, the pelvis is rotated by raising the buttocks from the floor. Muscular effort is required for this movement. As the buttocks are being raised, the lower back *must not be permitted to leave the floor.* Allowing the low back to arise from the floor would be equivalent to a "wrestler's bridge." This would result in *hyperextension* of the lumbar spine rather than in the reversal of lordosis caused by raising the buttocks while the lower back is pressed flat against the floor.

A helpful teaching tip is to place one hand on the symphysis pubic region, the other at the xiphoid process, and bring them together in the front, while the pelvis is elevated at the same time.

The patient is next taught slow rhythmic elevation of the pelvis with the lower back remaining *flat* against the floor. This permits smooth pelvic tilting which not only flattens the lumbar lordosis but gives the patient the kinesthetic concept of this tilting movement and simultaneously helps stretch the lower back. Endurance, as well as strength, is developed in the gluteal and abdominal muscles, which are the principal pelvic-tilting muscles (Fig. 28).

As the concept and the ability to flatten the back is achieved with the hips fully flexed the attempt should now be made to continue the tilting movement while the legs are gradually extended. As the legs ultimately become fully extended, the upright position, or its equivalent, is assumed. Flattening of the lower back becomes increasingly more difficult as the legs become more extended at the hips. Any degree of tightness or restriction of the hip flexors increases the difficulty in flattening the lower back (Fig. 29).

ABDOMINAL STRENGTHENING EXERCISES

In a study of the muscular mechanism by which the pelvis is tilted, it is obvious that strength and endurance must exist in the abdominal and gluteal muscles. It is tempting for the patient knowing this to proceed on his own to develop his abdominal muscles by the classical exercise of bilateral straight-leg raising done while in the supine position. Except in extremely athletic and physically well-conditioned individuals, this exercise is *contraindicated.*

In the supine position, with both legs fully extended, the first 30 degrees of straight-leg raising is done by the iliopsoas muscle. The kinesiology of the ilipsoas muscle is hip flexion. The psoas muscle attaches within the abdomen from the anterolateral aspect of the lumbar vertebrae and their transverse processes. This muscle bundle obliquely traverses the pelvis to attach to the lesser trochanter of the femur.

Contraction of the iliopsoas on the fixed lumbar spine results in flexion of the femur on the pelvis (Fig. 30). When the femur is fixed the converse occurs in that the psoas insertion becomes the origin, and the origin in turn becomes the insertion on the lumbar spine. Shortening of the muscle from the fixed femur causes traction on the anterior portion of the lumbar spine and results in increase in lumbar spine lordosis.

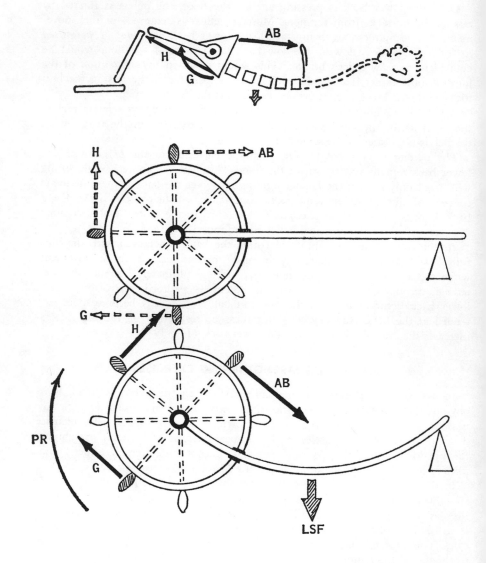

FIGURE 29. Direction of forces applied to pelvic rotation.
H   = Hamstring force
G   = Gluteal force
AB = Abdominal force
PR = Pelvic rotation
LSF = Lumbar spine flattening

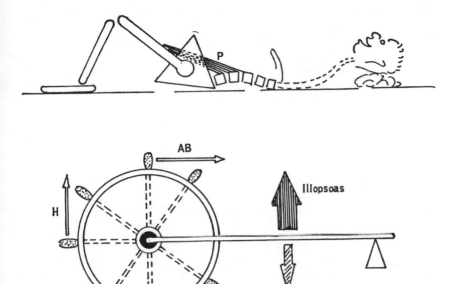

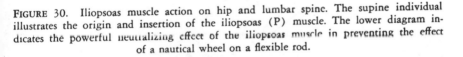

FIGURE 30. Iliopsoas muscle action on hip and lumbar spine. The supine individual illustrates the origin and insertion of the iliopsoas (P) muscle. The lower diagram indicates the powerful neutralizing effect of the iliopsoas muscle in preventing the effect of a nautical wheel on a flexible rod.

In view of the heaviness of the legs and the frequent weakness of the abdominal muscles, the first degrees of bilateral straight-leg raising cause the back to arch, and as a result the legs move very slightly. To this back-arching effect is added the intra-abdominal strain, plus the breath-holding Valsalva effect; therefore the contraindication to bilateral straight-leg raising from the supine position can be understood.

After 30 degrees or more of straight-leg raising, the iliopsoas becomes less effective in contraction and the abdominals become more efficient. From this position the pelvis will rotate and the lumbar spine flatten. If abdominal strengthening exercises are to be prescribed, they should begin when the legs have been raised to an angle of 30 degrees or when the hips and knees are flexed.

The *curl up* from the supine position, with the hips and knees flexed, is the second stage of abdominal-muscle strengthening. *Curl up* can be done from the supine position in which the head and shoulders are *peeled* up from the floor with a gradual curl to the point of having the nose touch the knees

(Fig. 31). This exercise requires strong abdominal muscles but may be done with the feet held down.

In the presence of significant weakness of the abdomen, this exercise can be done in reverse. The *curl up* exercise is done as an *uncurl* exercise. From the fully curled-up position, with nose to knees, the patient leans back slightly from his flexed knees. After a few degrees of *uncurling*, the patient returns to the full-curled position. Progressive uncurling with return to full flexed position is to be repeated until extension to the complete supine position and its return are possible.

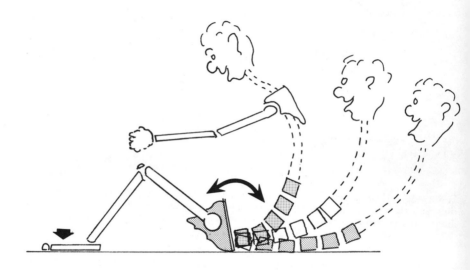

FIGURE 31. Abdominal strengthening exercise. With hips and knees flexed and the feet held down, "curl ups" are done in slow rhythmic manner. If there is weakness at first, the position of full flexion is used at the start; exercise consists of going back and forth until the individual is able to arise fully from complete supine position.

LOW BACK STRETCHING EXERCISES

A tight low back, or inflexible lumbar spine, will impede trunk flexion. This condition may have been discovered during the examination when the physician observed the patient bending forward from the upright position. Stretch pain elicited on flexing of the tight lower back may have been determined to be the cause of the low back pain. If the inelasticity of the low back is present and symptomatic, it must be made elastic or flexible. The lumbar-spinal longitudinal ligaments and muscles must be stretched to regain this elongation range.

Low back stretching is best done in the *curled-up-in-a-ball position*. The fetal, or knee to chest position, is attempted with the emphasis on having the patient feel that his lower back is being stretched. This can best be done by having the patient lie supine and rhythmically pull both knees back to his chest. It is not necessary, in fact it is usually not desirable, to raise the head from the floor. It certainly is not necessary to touch the knees with one's nose even if it is possible to do so. These added maneuvers at best may cause more straining than stretching.

It may be well to delay the rhythmical flexing of both legs to the chest and to substitute an exercise in which only one leg at a time is brought back to the chest. This is useful in attaining flexion limberness and is especially valuable when low back stretch pain is manifest. Each leg should be brought bent to chest ten times rhythmically. This should be followed by the exercise for both legs, repeated ten times, with the emphasis on the lower back being stretched. Such exercise usually suffices to elongate the back.

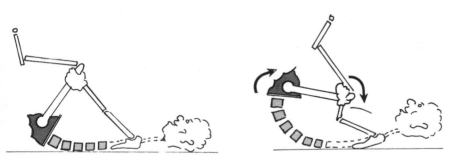

FIGURE 32. Low back stretching exercise. In the supine position, each knee is brought rhythmically and gently to the ipsilateral armpit. The knee is not to be brought to the nose nor vice versa. The thigh is used as a lever. The lower leg should not be forced against the thigh as this can force flex the knee.

A modification of the supine low-back stretch is the *yoga* position. The patient sits with both knees flexed towards the chest and with knees spread apart sufficiently to permit the body to bend down between the separated knees. The head is "bobbed" down towards the feet. The feet may be grasped by the hands, the elbows being between the legs, to permit the arms to help stretch the lower back. This exercise is more taxing than that of the supine knee-to-chest exercise and will require careful supervision and a slower gradual increase.

Any tendency to stretch the lower back by bending forward in an upright position with knees stiff, in a bouncing attempt to touch the toes with the fingers, should be avoided. This exercise can stretch the lower back but does so forcefully insofar as the hamstrings hold the pelvis fixed after a certain degree of rotation. The hamstrings, since they are less elastic and resilient than the lower part of the back, may cause a too violent low back stretch. The ability to touch one's toes with knees held straight is not a criterion of flexibility.

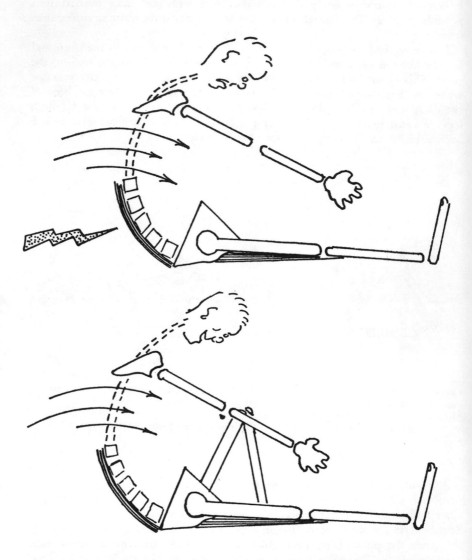

FIGURE 33. Protective hamstring stretching exercise. Upper picture depicts the method of stretching both hamstrings simultaneously, which results in overstretching the low back. The lower picture shows the pelvic immobilization by flexing one hip and then stretching the other hamstring.

HAMSTRING STRETCHING EXERCISES

If the presence of tight hamstrings is discovered during the observation of the *lumbar pelvic rhythm* kinetics, it is necessary that they be required to undergo stretching exercises. The inclination to stretch both hamstrings simultaneously by trying to bend forward at the trunk and keeping the legs extended may do harm, cause pain, and at best be ineffective as far as stretching the hamstrings is concerned. For this reason *protective* hamstring stretching is advocated (Fig. 33); the term *protective* implies that the low back is to be protected from excess stretching during the exercise.

The supine sitting position is used for the protective stretching exercise of the hamstring-muscle group. In such exercise the leg is fully flexed at the hip while the knee with the thigh is brought close to the chest; the foot in turn is placed flat against the floor. The leg undergoing the stretching exercise is extended straight ahead. Next, the flexed leg is rotated outward, and the knee is allowed to abduct. This action permits the patient to reach towards the toes of his extended leg. Reaching towards the toes is done in a bouncing rhythmical manner. The stretch sensation must be felt in the extended leg. The flexed leg prevents stretching of the low back, and thus no pain from stretching can occur in the low back.

It must be kept in mind that this exercise is aimed at stretching connective tissue and myostatic contracture. If, however, the unilateral stretch pain is due to an irritable sciatic nerve rather than to inelastic connective tissue, this exercise will not be beneficial. As a rule, unilateral stretch pain emanating from straight-leg raising, with no contralateral stretch pain, more frequently is sciatica rather than pain caused by stretching tight hamstrings.

HEEL CORD STRETCHING EXERCISES

When restrictive heel cords are found to impair body mechanics, they may be stretched during the course of the protective hamstring stretch-exercise by merely placing at a 90 degree angle the sole of the foot of the extended leg flat against a wall. The bouncing action which stretches the hamstring will simultaneously stretch the heel cord.

The heel cords may also be stretched effectively when the patient stands erect but leans forward against a wall. To take this position, the patient should stand a few feet away from the wall and stretch forward until the palms of his hands rest against the wall. In this position the body of the patient leans at an angle to the wall, but balanced on both feet and resting on both palms.

Once in this position, with *one* foot, the patient steps forward halfway to the wall. Keeping his other leg extended at the knee and the heel firmly on the ground, the patient then flexes rhythmically the forward leg at the knee. Flexing the arms allows a total back-and-forth movement of the entire body but the rear heel must be kept flat against the floor. In this way, a stretching effect is exerted on the heel cord (Fig. 34). Care must be taken during this

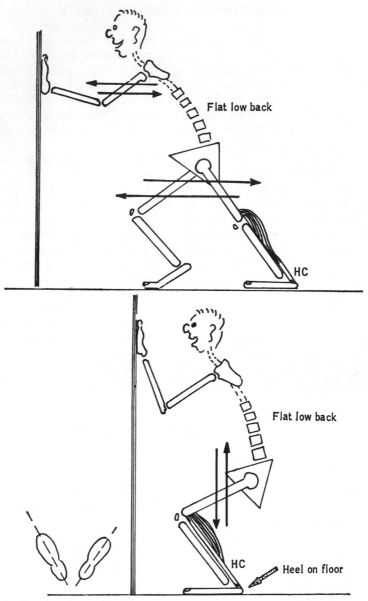

FIGURE 34. Exercises for heel cord stretching.

The upper diagram illustrates the manner of stretching a unilateral heel cord by leaning against a wall and moving back and forth. The rear foot is kept flat against the floor which insures stretching of the heel cord. The forward leg is flexed to permit to and fro rocking. The lumbar spine must be prevented from arching.

In the lower diagram, bilateral heel cord stretching is done by "squatting" and sitting on both heels. The feet are placed slightly apart and externally rotated. The stretching motion is a rhythmic up and down bounce with balance maintained against a wall or chair.

exercise to prevent arching of the lower region of the back as the leaning position against the wall is conducive to arching. A flat back must be maintained constantly.

A method of bilateral heel cord stretching may be suggested (Fig. 34, lower diagram) that appears exceedingly simple, yet cannot be performed by everyone. The person squats as if he intends to sit on his heels, and at the same time keeps both feet slightly turned out and several inches apart. Both heels must be kept on the floor and any use of the soles of the feet or toes must be avoided while a bouncing deep-knee bend is performed. In assuming the position necessary for this exercise the person will naturally feel the stretching taking place in heel cords. Because this exercise may place a person off balance, it should be done with support from a chair or wall.

EXERCISES FOR STRETCHING HIP FLEXORS

Stretching of tight hip flexors (the iliopsoas group) is a difficult exercise. The hip flexors are difficult to isolate and the stretching of hip flexors without simultaneously hyperextending the lumbar spine takes a concentrated effort; frequently it requires assistance. The correct stretching of this muscle group presupposes that the patient has mastered pelvic tilting and therefore is capable of maintaining a flat back during the exercise.

This exercise can be performed in several ways. One of them is done in the supine position with the extended leg held down against the floor. The extended leg is the one in which the hip flexor is to be stretched. This leg can be held down by placing the leg under a bed or sofa, by using a heavy sandbag, or by having another person render assistance. The opposite leg is then flexed rhythmically to the chest as in the knee-chest exercise (Fig. 35, upper diagram).

As the flexed leg is brought repeatedly to the chest, the hip flexors of the opposite leg receive the benefit of the exercise.

In another form of the exercise, the patient may lie supine on a table or bed and dangle one leg from the table. The weight of the dangling leg will then come into play to stretch the hip flexor. In this exercise there will also occur the stretching of the quadriceps femoris which may be prevented by reducing the degree of knee flexion of the dangling leg. The remainder of this exercise is done in the same manner as when it is performed on the floor.

The hip flexors may also be stretched by a position in which the patient kneels on only one knee (Fig. 35, lower diagram). It is in this leg that the pelvis becomes extended and thus causes that hip flexor to be stretched. The forward leg is to be flexed at the hip and knee, the foot being kept on the floor. A rocking motion forward and backwards of the entire body while in this position will result in the desired stretching of the flexor hip group.

Exercises to flatten the lower back, and methods of stretching the tissues that conceivably could restrict mobility have been discussed. Subsequently, the application of this newly acquired pelvic movement and the tissue flexibility into practical kinetic functioning must follow.

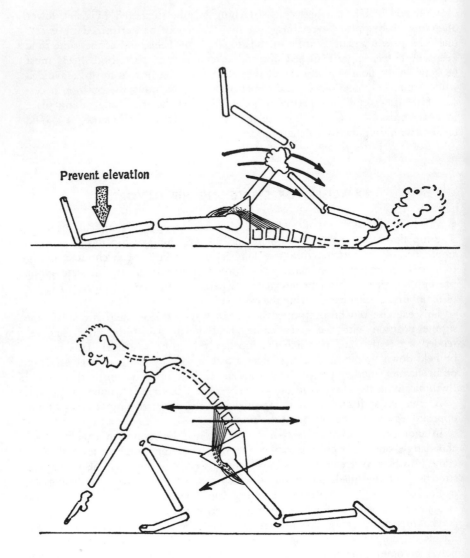

Prevent elevation

FIGURE 35. Exercises for stretching the hip flexors.

Upper diagram illustrates a manner of stretching unilateral hip flexors described in the text. The extended leg is held down in several ways and the lumbar spine must explicitly be prevented from arching.

As shown in the lower diagram, the kneeling method of stretching hip flexor is done in a to and fro rocking rhythm and the flexed hip anchors the pelvis and maintains a flexed lumbar spine.

LUMBAR-PELVIC RHYTHM TRAINING

Performance of pelvic tilting learned in the supine position should now be learned in the upright position. This exercise may be done by using a wall as the floor was used in the supine pelvic-tilting exercises. The person should be directed to lean back against a wall with the feet some 12 to 18 inches from the wall. This will permit flattening of the lower part of the back against a firm surface. In this way, pelvic-tilting exercises done in the supine position are now done with the patient upright against the wall.

In the process of this exercise, as the back begins to flatten out with less effort, the feet are gradually brought closer to the baseboard of the wall. The same effect may be achieved when the hips and knees are merely flexed while the lower back is continued to be pressed against the wall. In this position the knees are gradually straightened. Both of these modifications permit the same desired result of flattening the lower-back curve when the person finally takes an upright-erect position. This upright position against a supporting wall is the goal of proper posture. When this stance can be performed unsupported, the ultimate object of proper posture has been reached.

A *flat back* is so designated because the lumbosacral angle is decreased and the lumbar spine is less curved. There is less shearing stress of L_5 on S_1, L_4 on L_5 and in the others in the sequence. The posterior articulations are separated by this posture and accordingly are less subject to weight bearing. Less ligamentous strain is imposed and consequently better balance exists between muscle tone and ligamentous balance. All these factors insure less fatigue because of a better balanced spine.

Flat back posture fulfills the definition of correct body posture as described in the work "Posture and Its Relationship to Orthopedic Disabilities" by the Posture Committee of the American Academy of Orthopedic Surgeons in 1947.

"Posture is usually defined as the relative arrangement of the parts of the body. Good posture is the state of muscular and skeletal balance which protects the supporting structures of the body against injury or progressive deformity irrespective of the attitude (erect, lying, squatting, stooping) in which these structures are working or resting. Under such conditions the muscles will function most efficiently and the optimum positions are afforded for the thoracic and abdominal organs. Poor posture is a faulty relationship of the various parts of the body which produce increased strain on the supporting structures and in which there is less efficient balance of the body over the base of support."

Likewise, in any kinetic operation of the body, a similarly balanced relationship of the parts to each other must remain to insure minimal strain and minimal muscular effort. Hence, during movement a flat back balanced over the plumb-line center of gravity should be maintained.

When the patient bends forward, the lumbar curve must reverse. It is necessary that the patient should learn to bend with his knees slightly flexed. In this way, the hamstrings are relaxed and, therefore, impose less restriction on pelvic rotation. This affords less occasion for forcing flexion of the lumbar spine beyond its physiologic limits.

For the person who must remain in a partially bent position during long

71

periods of the day, such as the barber, dentist, or housewife who works over a sink or a crib, less fatigue will result from such posture if the back is kept flat and the center of gravity maintained over the hips and feet. No discomfort occurs in the absence of ligamentous strain.

Flexing one hip will help in assuming flat back posture by releasing hip-flexor pull on the lumbar spine. Thus, placing one foot on a small stool with the knee and hip flexed will permit an upright position with less lumbar lordosis (Fig. 36).

In everyday activities one must always keep in mind the benefit of a low back kept *flat*. In addition, all the tissues having a stressful reaction on the spine are kept inoperative. For example, neutral position of sitting erect in a pain-free effortless attitude requires a chair with a firm seat and back. The

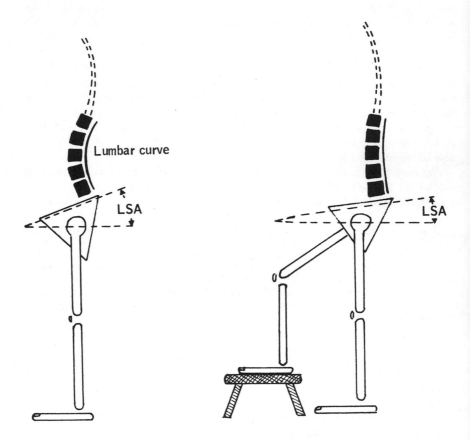

FIGURE 36. Relaxed prolonged standing posture. A small stool for one foot flexes the hip of that leg and thus relaxes the iliopsoas and "flattens" the lumbar curve. This method is advisable for dentists, housewives, barbers, etc.

height of the seat should permit the legs to be flexed free at the knees. The base of the spine should rest merely a few inches forward of the chair back. The feet should reach the floor from a seat height that supports the thighs. When the rest of the chair is high, the feet may dangle placing pressure on the posterior thigh area and disrupt a relaxed pelvic balance. Too low a chair seat increases the hip flexor angle and forces a person to bend forward upon his pelvis. The chair back should offer firm contact for the spine 4 to 6 inches above the seat and an area of contact with the upper lumbar spine and the lower thoracic spine. This firm, flat chair-back permits the lumbar spine to be erect but prevents a fatiguing stance that is flexed so much it causes prolonged ligamentous strain.

In Fig. 37 proper chair-sitting posture is illustrated in A. In the secretarial chair depicted in B, the support for the small of the back is too high and too narrow. The point of low-back contact is at the mid-lumbar point, forcing the spine to arch around this pressure fulcrum. The rotation of the pelvis resulting from this increased lordosis places a stretch strain on the hamstring muscles. The conflict between the hamstring pull and low-back arch terminates in fatigue and pain.

The automobile seat or the soft, deep sofa places an elongation hamstring pull on the pelvis with a resultant flexion on the lumbar spine that exceeds the flat lumbar curve. Pain in this instance arises from hamstring stretch and concurrent low-back posterior-longitudinal ligamentous strain.

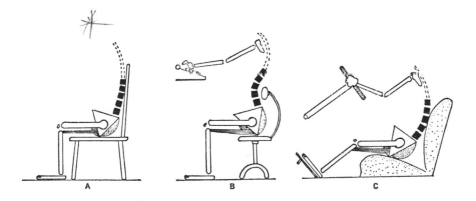

FIGURE 37. Sitting postures. A, Correct sitting posture in a firm straight-back chair in which seat has the proper width and height to allow hips and knee to be flexed with no strain and both feet touching the floor. The back of the chair supports the low back 4 to 6 inches from the seat and permits a "flat" lumbar curve.

B, The chair back increases the arch and causes a hamstring strain and a fatiguing low back posture.

C, The hamstrings are taut and place traction on the pelvis, causing rotation and ultimately strain on the low back.

73

The major kinetic stress on the spine occurs during the reversing of the lumbar-pelvic rhythm when the body returns to the erect from the bent-over position. In bending forward the lumbar spine has flexed to its full capability, and the pelvis that has fully rotated in a rhythmical manner must now return to the erect position, but this action must be performed in a similar rhythmic manner. In other words, gradual return of the lumbar lordosis must be synchronously accompanied by gradual rotation of the pelvis to its erect static angle. The proper manner of assuming the erect position is to tuck in the pelvis on reassuming the erect from the bent-over posture. This same procedure is to be followed when the sitting position is changed to the erect. "Tuck in" is the vernacular term for rotation of the pelvis, an action in which the anterior portion is elevated and the sacral portion is depressed. This motion brings the buttocks *under* the low back. Slight bending of the knees can aid this tucking in of the pelvis. Lifting a heavy object or a bulky object must be done not only with the strength of the knees but with the pelvis tucked in while at the same time the lifted object is held close to the body. Lifting an object with the help of the knees and with an arched back fails to protect the lower area of the back. Tucking in the pelvis is the key to normal back movement (Fig. 38).

A simple means of maintaining a flat low-back while the body is in an erect position is to place an object between the buttocks and "squeeze" the object. This "squeezing" is essentially gluteus maximus contraction—a muscular action that tilts the pelvis. This concept of "squeezing" and the subsequent tilting can readily be sensed by the patient. "Squeezing" can be practiced on an imaginary object, such as a coin placed between the buttocks. If in all positions and activities a person will remember to "squeeze" this imaginary coin, proper static and kinetic posture and function will be assured.

LATERAL FLEXIBILITY EXERCISE

A laterally oblique pelvis from which the spine takes off at right angle and curves laterally to resume vertical level must be corrected if the obliquity is marked. Pelvic obliquity from a short leg can be corrected by shoe correction. After the correction has been made to insure proper leg length which in turn levels off the pelvis area, the compensatory lateral lumbar curve may simultaneously correct itself. Once the pelvis is level, the spine should be straight. To permit this compensatory straightening, the spine must have lateral flexibility to both sides, left and right.

If, however, the laterally curving spine, which is assumed to be compensating for the oblique pelvis, is not flexible, merely raising or lengthening one leg will not correct the spinal alignment and consequently will not re-align the posterior facet articulations. An inflexible lateral "C" curve of the spine caused by an oblique pelvis must be assumed to be inflexible because of an adaptive myostatic contracture and contracted pericapsular and ligamentous tissues. These tissues must be stretched before a leg-length correction will be of func-

74

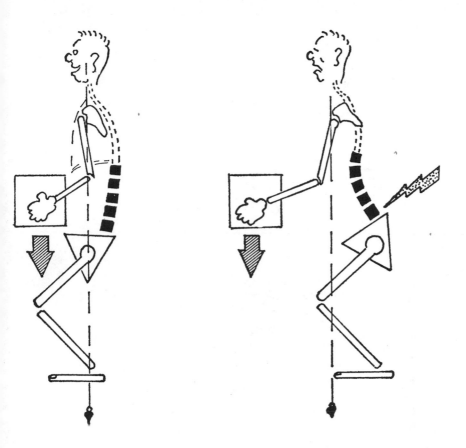

FIGURE 38. Correct and incorrect method of lifting.

The correct manner of lifting is shown in the picture to the left in that the object is held close to the body, the pelvis is "tucked in" under the flattened lumbar spine and the effort of lifting is delegated to the hip and knee extensors.

The incorrect manner, in spite of lifting "with the legs," shows the back arched and the object at a distance from the body. The "lever arm" principle of these mechanisms has been discussed in Figure 23.

tional value. The bone changes of a prolonged scoliosis will not be corrected, but at least the periarticular and ligamentous tissue can be stretched.

Stretching is best done with the patient in upright position while the pelvis is tucked in and slightly flexed. Lateral stretching of the lumbar spine with the back arched is anatomically impossible. Extension of the lumbar spine approximates the posterior facets and in their almost pure vertical plane permits no significant lateral nor rotary movement. Some lateral movement is possible in the flexed spine. The lateral trunk stretching exercise is explained in the

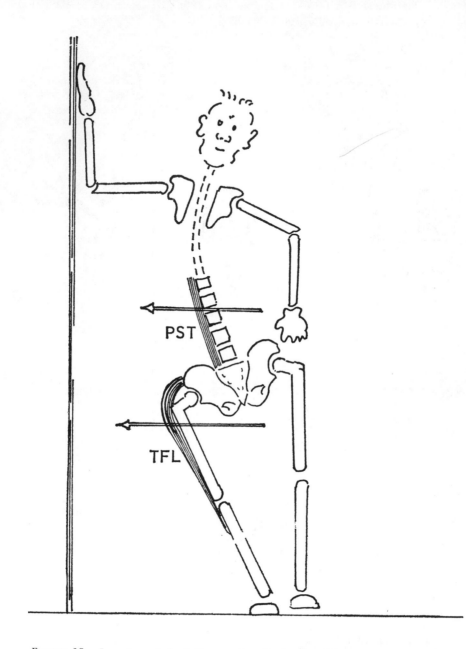

FIGURE 39. Lateral trunk flexibility exercises. By leaning sideways against a wall with both feet sufficiently far from the wall to shift the center of gravity the spine will laterally bend towards the wall. The paraspinous tissues (PST) towards the wall, on the convex spinal side will be stretched. The Tensor fascia lata (TFL) on that side nearest the wall will also be stretched during this exercise.

caption for Figure 39. This exercise, done primarily for lateral trunk flexibility, simultaneously stretches the tensor fascia lata. Tightness of the tensor fascia lata frequently accompanies the presence of a short leg.

A lateral "C" curve, not due to a pelvic obliquity, may imply a structural curve rather than an adaptive functional curve. Lateral stretching of a structural curvature will not greatly increase lateral flexibility. A heel lift to correct a short leg condition will also benefit a structural curve, but obviously to a lesser degree. The response, though admittedly less in a structural scoliosis, should be beneficial and such exercise therefore is advised.

A lateral lumbar curve existing within a shorter segmental level as part of an "S" scoliosis is probably structural and will be present irrespective of a concomitant pelvic obliquity. Lateral stretch here also will yield only limited gain in lateral range but the gain in flexibility is always justified and beneficial. A heel lift should aid in maintaining the erectness and flexibility acquired by the flexibility exercises. X-ray studies may be required to differentiate a structural from a functional scoliosis. Exercises intelligently done can but do good regardless of the etiology of the curve.

SUMMARY

As established from the history and physical examination, the treatment of the mechanical low-back pain is based on the correction of faulty *static* posture and faulty *kinetic* mechanism of the lumbar spine.

Static abnormalities are essentially the result of faulty posture, and correction of these faults with resultant good posture should result in a pain-free stance. Adequate flexibility, good muscle tone, and proper concept of good kinesthetics are essential for the maintenance of proper posture.

Proper *kinetic* function requires adequate flexibility of all movement components involved in the performance of correct *lumbar-pelvic rhythm*. All the components concerned in the rhythm must function correctly. Insofar as movement requires muscular effort, sometimes strength, and sometimes endurance, and at times both, good muscle conditioning is paramount. All factors composing the kinetic function must be adequate and must be organized in a facile and almost automatic functional pattern. Exercises will achieve maximum flexibility and produce maximum muscle strength and endurance. Proper performance constantly practiced will result in everyday function free of pain owing to the proper use of a properly conditioned machine.

Disk Disease

Disk disease today is the object of wide discussion as a specific disease entity; yet its origin and presence do not enjoy conformity of interpretation. The terms disk *degeneration, rupture, slipping, bulging* are used interchangeably as if their significance were the same; yet such terms avoid accurate functional definition

Much is known concerning disk anatomy and chemistry. The physiology of the disk is becoming understood and its pathophysiology has been defined. Sufficient knowledge is held today to interpret its normal mechanical function so that it is possible to evaluate its deviation from normal. This recognition permits a rational therapeutic approach.

The intervertebral disk is a hydraulic system composed of a fibroelastic cylinder containing a colloidal gel. The disks compose one quarter of the supporting spine structure of the human body and are constantly exposed to compression, torque, and shearing stresses. These tissues under repeated stresses over the years are subject to degeneration from wear and tear. Such degeneration can lead to impaired function and morbidity.

DEGENERATIVE CHANGES

The elasticity of the annulus is dependent upon the changes in the direction of the intertwining fibers. As degeneration occurs, because of aging or repeated trauma, the collagenous rings lose their intactness and become fragmented. Mechanical stress imposed upon this fragmented annulus will force an infiltration of mucoid tissue out through these rents into the interstices. Ultimately this extruded mucoid material will be contained merely within the confines of the outer fibrous capsule.

The annulus is weakest in its posterior lateral aspect, and this region is the commonest site of bulging or herniation. Because the posterior longitudinal ligament is incomplete in the lower lumbar area it also permits an easier site for hernia to manifest itself (Fig. 40). The posterior longitudinal ligament is complete throughout the length of the spine but upon reaching the L_1 level on its caudal descent it tapers off and at its attachment on S_1 is only partial, covering only 50 per cent of the posterior disk space.

Aging decreases the elastic qualities of the intervertebral disks, but this aging of itself does not constitute disk disease. The mere aging process need not contribute to morbidity and pain if all other factors in the spine physiology are adequate.

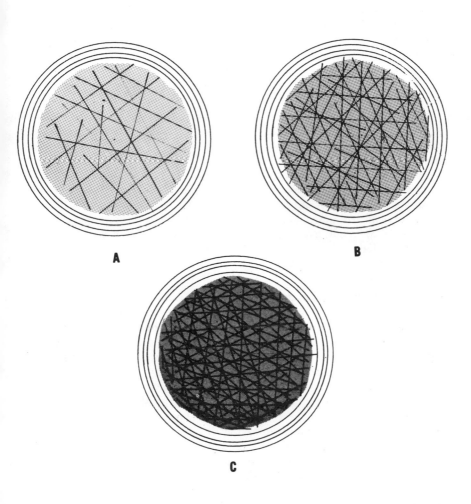

FIGURE 40.   Intervertebral disk nucleus degeneration.

A, The young normal nucleus with a homogeneous matrix embedded in ultramicroscopic fibrils.

B, With aging there is dehydration of the matrix and increase in thickness of the fibrils.

C, With further aging, the nucleus is a firm fibrous shrunken mass with very little water content.

79

A constitutional variant must be considered to exist in some disks that predispose them to earlier degeneration than others. Numerous traumata also must play a significant role. Every stress applied to the disk can theoretically cause some tearing and fragmentation of the fibroelastic annulus. Every tear in the annulus is replaced by fibrous tissue rather than by elastic fibrils, and any colloidal gel that leaks out is replaced by a colloid having less imbibitory qualities.

The significance of shearing stress imposing major strain on disks is evident in the relatively high incidence of degeneration at the lumbosacral junction manifest at L_5-S_1 and in the cervical spine at C_{5-6} and C_{6-7}. Both of these sites of degeneration are to be found at the apices of curvature and spine angulation. Poor posture increases this angulation and mechanically permits added shearing stress. Increase in angulation is evident in excessive lumbar lordosis. In the cervical spine the compensatory increase in cervical lordosis to compensate for a dorsal kyphosis has a similar mechanical effect. It must also be remembered that the maximum movement of total spinal flexion and extension occurs at the lumbosacral (L_5-S_1) joint and, incidentally, in the neck at the C_{5-6} and C_{6-7} levels.

Poor body conditioning contributes a significant part to disk degeneration. Insofar as disk nutrition is considered to be by imbibition, the nutrients must be brought to the disk by adequate circulation. The surrounding tissue must be maintained sufficiently flexible to permit tissue-fluid effusion and diffusion. Good muscle tone and contractility are essential in supplying suitable circulation to the region.

COMPRESSION AND TENSION EFFECTS ON DISKS

Gravity imposes a strain on the elastic shock-absorbing weight-bearing disks. The upright erect position of itself imposes daily stress. This strain is compressive in contradistinction to the shearing stress previously discussed. The superiority of recumbency as a means of decreasing compressive strain on the disk is obvious.

Brief compression loads imposed upon the normal disk may cause distortion of the disk but no permanent deformity. Deformity is greater in the degenerated disk. Constant pressure on the disk whether sustained or recurrent plays a substantial degenerating role. Tension when repeated or prolonged must therefore be considered a straining and damaging force on the disk.

The term *tension* needs qualification. Physical tension in which the body muscles are sustained in a state of isometric contraction exerts a vise-like pressure on the disk that ultimately decreases its imbibitory faculty. The disk under this tension force is maintained in a static state of compression. It may be compared to the squeezed sponge that cannot absorb water until it is released and permitted to expand. In addition to the compression of the disk, the contracted muscles do not perform their massaging effect and therefore do not bring fresh blood to the part, nor do the contracted muscles carry away from the area the "used" blood. Virtual stagnation exists.

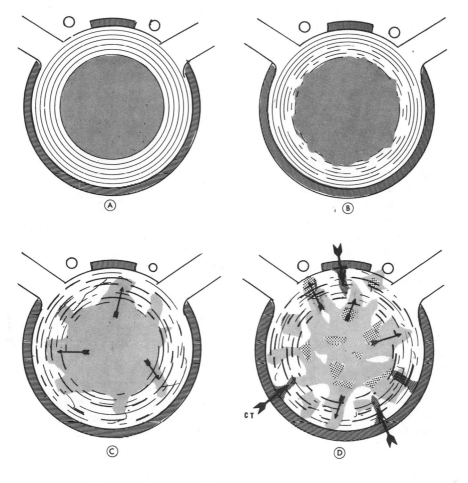

FIGURE 41. Degenerative changes in the intervertebral disk.

A, The normal young disk.

B, The nucleus shows beginning dehydration and there are already some tears and fragmentation in the annulus.

C, More advanced changes than in B with nuclear material escaping outward into the annular tears.

D, Repair process in which connective tissue, CT, invades inward carrying blood vessels, fibroblasts, nerves, etc.

81

Tension as described above is noted in sustained muscular contraction during the performance of a physical act. Such tension exists in the performance of heavy weight-lifting and also in the performance of a tedious task requiring prolonged fine-point concentration.

Emotional tension, through its somatic muscular component, imposes equal muscular tension in addition to the sustained muscular contraction of physical work. Sustained isometric muscular contraction imposed on the body by the nervous tense irritable person and which is unrelieved by periods of relaxation acts similiar to the vise-like effect of physical tension.

SPONDYLOSIS

The disease entity of *degenerative arthritis* of the spine is a sequela to intervertebral disk degeneration. Degenerative arthritis, hypertrophic arthritis, discogenic degenerative disease, osteoarthropathy, and spondylosis are morbidly and mechanically similar, toward which disk degeneration is undoubtedly a predisposing factor.

As the disk degenerates, the elastic fibers of the annulus decrease and are replaced by fibrous tissue. A loss of elasticity ensues, and flexibility of movement between two vertebrae is diminished. The intradiskal pressure that normally assists in keeping the vertebrae apart is decreased, and the vertebrae approximate. Shock-absorbing ability is decreased. The fibrous capsule and its ligaments become slack, and anterior-posterior shearing movement, normally not possible, can now occur.

Two pathologic conditions, capable of causing pain, result. The ligaments slacken when the vertebrae approximate, vertebral periosteal attachment of the ligaments weakens, and any pressure exerted on the ligament permits a dissection away from its periosteal attachment. Disk material usually confined within a taut ligamentous compartment can now dissect the slack ligament from its previous site of attachment on the vertebrae (Fig. 41). Further extrusion of disk material is facilitated by the fragmentation of the annulus.

The material extruded decreases the quantity of disk tissue between the vertebrae and permits further vertebral approximation, further ligamentous laxity, more dissection of the ligamentous-periosteal attachment, and further protrusion of nuclear material: the process becomes a vicious cycle. The extruded material, since it is a foreign body, evokes an irritation reaction. This irritation may be removed by fibrous replacement followed by calcification. This calcified extruded tissue becomes the "arthritic spur" seen on x-ray film. Because of this the concept of spondylosis evolution appears feasible (Fig. 42).

ACUTE AND CHRONIC ARTICULAR SYNOVITIS

Another pathologic condition resulting from the narrowing of the disk space ensues in the posterior articulations. Narrowing of the disk in the anterior weight-bearing portion permits approximation of the vertebral bodies. As the

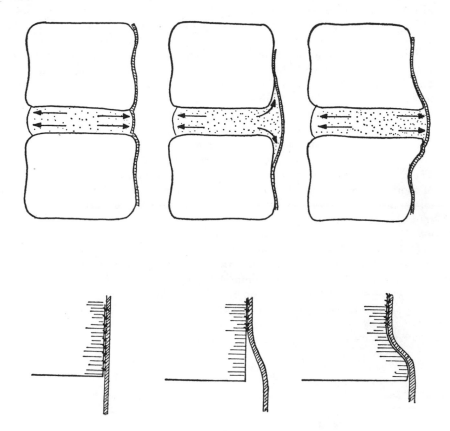

FIGURE 42. Mechanism of spondylosis.

A, The normal anterior portion of the functional unit with an intact disk, normal interspace, and a taut posterior longitudinal ligament that is totally adherent to the vertebral body periosteum.

B, Disk degeneration permits approximation of the two vertebrae causing a slack in the posterior longitudinal ligament and intradiskal pressure permits dissection between periosteum and ligament.

C, The extruded disk material becomes fibrous then ultimately calcifies into what becomes a "spur."

vertebral bodies approximate anteriorly, the posterior articulation also reapproaches which changes the alignment of the facet surfaces. This facet malalignment places a strain on the synovial tissues of the facets and on the articular capsules. There is concurrently then less freedom of movement in the act of extension, and impingement of the opposing facets can occur more easily.

The combination of these two pathologic factors, namely, the anterior-vertebral approximation with its accompanying ligamentous bulging and the posterior-articular approximation of the facets encroaches upon and narrows the intervertebral foramen. This encroachment arises because of the approximation above and below of the two pedicles, anteriorly by the bulging longitudinal ligament and possibly early spur formation, and posteriorly by the encroaching facets and their swollen synovial capsule (Fig. 43).

Since the nerve root now emerges through a decreased foramen, it may be compressed. Extension of the spine increase the lumbar lordosis, further approximates the posterior articulations and thus narrows the intervertebral foraminal aperture. The mechanism of nerve root irritation ("sciatica") caused by spondylosis and aggravated by lumbar spine hyperextension in the presence of disk degeneration gives a clear picture of its own condition.

At this point the mechanism of nerve root irritation is understood by the doctor and the symptoms can be reproduced by a specific movement or position. The discovery alone of spurs on x-ray film is not sufficient. An x-ray diagnosis of spurs or degenerative arthritis is *not* synonymous with a clinical diagnosis of symptomatic spondylosis. Subjective sciatica admittedly can arise from nerve root pressure alone; in itself it may be insufficient to cause *objective* loss of motor, sensory, or reflex function.

Disk disease, disk degeneration, and spondylosis are similar terms and yet are not interchangeable. Understanding the meaning of the term itself is not as important as is the need for comprehending the mechanism. Another aspect of disk disease is disk "rupture" or lumbar disk "herniation." These two terms imply similar mechano-pathologic conditions.

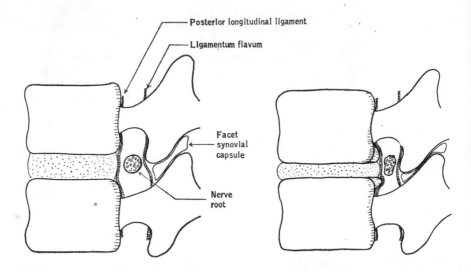

FIGURE 43. Intervertebral foraminal impingement in disk degeneration and spondylosis. The figure on the left shows the normal relationship of two vertebrae adequately separated by a normal disk. The foramen is open and the emerging nerve root free. The figure to the right depicts the foraminal narrowing due to osteophyte impingement and posterior articular closure with synovial irritation. Movement is obviously restricted and further nerve root pinch can be pictured by extension of this functional unit.

84

LUMBAR DISK HERNIATION

Disk herniation is fundamentally a release of the nuclear material from the confinement of the enveloping annulus fibrosus capsule. Herniation of the nuclear material may result from excessive forces, repeated stresses, and prolonged tension on the hydraulic mechanism or the presence of a faulty annulus, but any combination of the above may be involved. The formula previously mentioned may be applied here and the solution sought for in: (1) abnormal stress on normal mechanism, (2) normal stress on an abnormal mechanism, or (3) normal stress on a normal mechanism when the mechanism is not prepared to accept the stress.

Lumbar disk herniation is unequivocably a specific disease entity. The term *herniation*, or *rupture*, is more explainable and understandable in a mechanical sense than the term *slipped*. *Bulging* of the disk is also an accepted term. It is sufficient to say that the term used is of less importance than the realization of what is happening. It is much more significant to know the *where* and *what* of the disk herniation that is causing the symptoms, the *why* of the consequent treatment, and the *when* if there is a need for surgical intervention. The *why* or the course of the disk rupture is not yet understood fully.

Symptoms

Clinically, the patient with a herniated lumbar disk presents a history of sciatica, pain running down his leg, originating either in the region of the low back or the buttocks. A history of an immediate preceding trauma, a fall, a blow, or an incident of heavy lifting need not be elicited. In fact, the immediate relationship of stress and the onset of pain is infrequent. The strain or repeated stresses have frequently occurred prior to the acute onset and have set the stage for the ultimate herniation. By *setting the stage* is meant the weakening of the annulus fibrosus which diminishes the elastic recoil against a stress. A minimal stress applied on the disk that is contained within a weakened defective annulus may cause the nuclear material to herniate (Fig. 41).

The onset of sciatica ordinarily is abrupt. Pain most frequently begins as a low back pain, which usually is situated in the region of the lumbosacral spine but according to the patient's complaint it may run across the whole low-back or may restrict itself to one side of the lower region of back. As a rule, the pain initiates a sufficient spasm that immobilizes trunk function. As a result, the patient is unable to bend or to arise to a full erect position without evoking some degree of discomfort. Any movement of the trunk initiates spasm and pain.

In a large percentage of patients pain in the lower area of the back is felt simultaneously along the leg. Localizing such pain is of great diagnostic value. Pain, or the sensation of spasm, felt in the anterior thigh region, and usually perceived in both thighs is due to iliopsoas spasm which accompanies the acute scoliosis. This spasm is part of the immobilizing mechanism that prevents spine movement and actually splints the spine "away" from the site of irritation.

Sciatic pain, which is pressure neuritis, is a pain due to nerve irritation and the sensation is referred down the leg. The usual distribution of this pain referral is in the posterior thigh, the calf, heel, and into the toes. The patient's description actually points out to the examiner the specific nerve, and the extent to which it is being stressed.

Pain, described during the history taking actually classifies three circumstances for the doctor: *when* the pain is present; *what* aggravates it; and *what* relieves it. The *what* pertains to position or activity, and the *when* signifies type of related inciting activity, the time of day, its occurrence during period of strain or its association with fatigue. The *where* designates the origin of the pain and the part of the leg, foot, or toes affected by the irritation.

Mechanism

The mechanism by which the herniation of a lumbar disk causes symptoms of low back pain and sciatica is reasonably well understood. The biology and the chemical pathology of the disk remains obscure. The immediate pain in the back that usually is felt following herniation of a lumbar disk is probably due

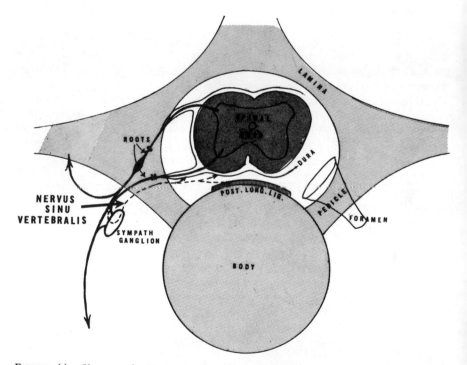

FIGURE 44. Sinu vertebralis nerve. The recurrent nerve of Luschka is considered to convey sensory fibers to the posterior longitudinal ligament, the dura, and reaching to the outer border of the annulus.

to irritation of the posterior longitudinal ligament which has been shown to be well supplied by sensory nerve fibers. The ligament is innervated by the sinu vertebralis nerve (the recurrent meningeal nerve, the recurrent nerve of Luschka) (Fig. 44).

Low back pain may also occur from irritation of the dural sleeve that accompanies the nerve root as it enters the intervertebral foramen. The posterior primary ramus goes to the posterior erector spinae muscles and can also account for the low back pain due to "muscle spasm."

If the disk herniates in a posterolateral direction, it can compress the nerve as it passes by the intervertebral disk on its way through the foramen. As the nerve root leaves the dural sac, it carries with it a *sleeve* of dura (Fig. 45).

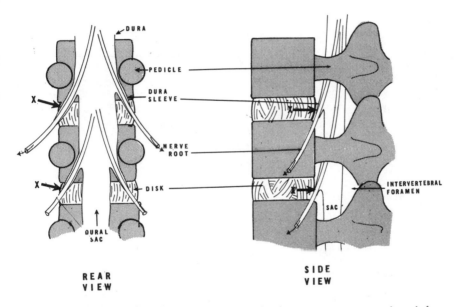

FIGURE 45. Dural sleeves of the nerve roots. As the nerve roots move lateral from the dural sac they carry a sleeve of dura through the intervertebral foramen. They pass near the disk in this posterior lateral region, and it is here that they can be compressed by a disk herniation.

This sleeve accompanies the nerve into the foramen but ends at its outer opening. At the point where the nerve penetrates the dura to form the sleeve, the sleeve is firmly attached and immovable. The dural sleeve is also firmly attached where it terminates at the outer opening of the foramen. Between these two points the dura can move very little and thus does not permit movement of itself or the enclosed nerve root away from any encroachment by a disk herniation.

Only at this posterolateral region of the intervertebral disk is the nerve in contact with it. Only here can disk herniation cause nerve root irritation and compression. Only by herniation in this region and direction can the symptoms and signs of sciatica be manifested.

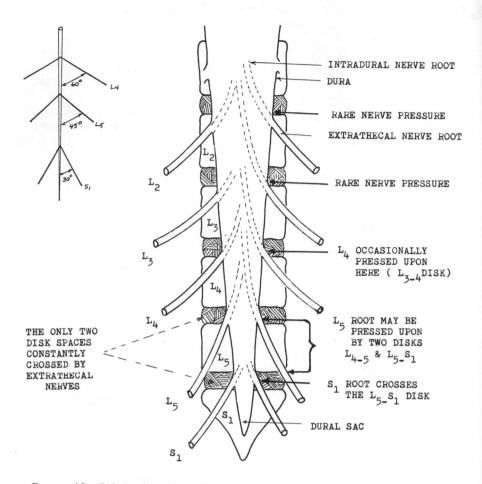

FIGURE 46. Relationship of specific nerve root to corresponding intervertebral disk.

Pain down the leg (so-called "sciatica") is related to the specific nerve root that is irritated. Each nerve involved has a specific sensory and motor distribution (Fig. 46). How far down the patient's leg the pain or numbness extends is considered dependent on the extent of pressure on the nerve by the intervertebral disk (Fig. 47).

The patient's history of the onset of disk herniation is not always a precise *cause and effect* story. A severe stress may have immediately preceded the onset of low back and leg pain, but often the immediate stress is mild or not even recalled. There may be a past history of recurrent mild and brief attacks of low back pain, with or without radiation into the leg. Previous attacks may have been severe, requiring days or weeks of bed rest or hospitalization. The

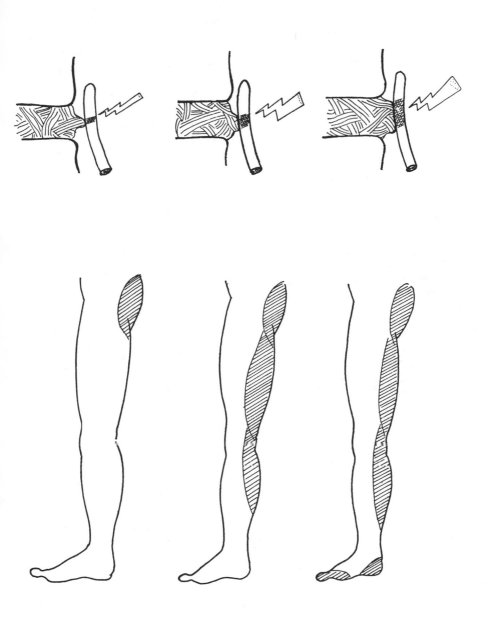

FIGURE 47. Subjective area of referred pain: correlation with area of nerve contact.

A, A slight degree of nerve contact will cause patient to claim pain referred to region of buttocks.

B, Pain claimed to radiate down posterior thigh, with or without buttocks pain, implies a greater degree of nerve contact.

C, Pain referred to the foot region implies a larger area of nerve contact and also gives an indication of the root spinal level. The amount of pressure is not so important as is the extent of the nerve contact at the foraminal level.

patient may recall that these attacks caused him to be "twisted to one side" (scoliosis, see Fig. 54), bent forward (the antalgic position, Fig. 53), or unable to stand fully erect. The pain was aggravated by bending, coughing, or sneezing. All these signs and symptoms imply previous nerve root irritation, probably due to disk herniation.

In very early life, by the age of fifteen, circumferential tears are noted in the annulus. They are discrete at first and found mostly near the nucleus (Fig. 48). As the years progress these concentric tears increase in number and extent. They tend to merge with others and ultimately are found in the outer margins of the annulus. They are asymptomatic and are considered to be an "ungluing" of the lamellae as the matrix dries up. It is evident that these "tears" are capable of weakening the annulus.

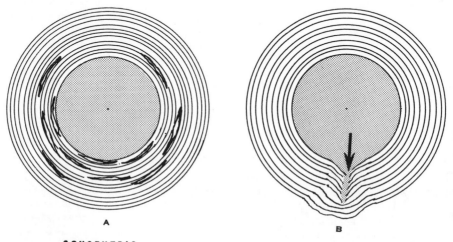

A   B

CONCENTRIC   RADIAL

FIGURE 48.   Annular changes in the aging disk.
A reveals concentric tears in the annulus that are first noted at age 15. They originate near the nucleus and are at first discrete. As the patient ages, they are found in greater number in the outer margin and tend to merge into larger tears.
B depicts radial tears. These too begin centrally and proceed outward. They are more numerous in the posterior portion of the disk. The pressure of the disk matrix pushes the torn fiber margins outward. When they reach the outer margin they "bulge" and deform the disk.

As aging and repeated trauma occurs, *radial* tears appear in the annulus (Fig. 48). These begin centrally near the nucleus and progress outwardly. Due to the pressure within the nucleus, the torn ends of the fibers are forced outwardly. When these tears reach the outer margin of the lamellae they can produce a "bulge." These radial tears deform the disk and impair its hydraulic properties, causing an increased mobility of the adjacent vertebra and thus instability. The concentric tears and radial tears occur more frequently in the posterior aspect of the annulus where their presence has obvious clinical significance.

90

Each episode of trauma has apparently set the stage for ultimate extrusion of the nucleus into the annular tears. Now a minor stress can "tip the scales." Occasionally the precipitating episode is severe and pain follows immediately. Most patients, however, recall only a minor strain followed by symptoms of low back pain and nerve root irritation. A sequence of mild strains initiating severe symptoms leads to the frequent controversy of *cause and effect* in medicolegal decisions and in dispositions of industrial injury claims.

In the evolution of the mechanism of disk herniation, the various factors elicited in the history can be correlated. Repeated minor traumata, with no sciatic radiation but with resultant low back pains, may well have been the episodes that gradually weakened the annulus. These repeated strains may be a series of strains from the lifting of heavy objects or may be acute facet impingements from minor physical activities. They may have been innocuous lifting or bending incidents but there was a mild structural back defect in the person who performed them. All of these have the ability to set the stage for ultimate disk herniation producing subjective and objective signs and symptoms.

Diagnosis

The onset of the pain may be related to the back alone or exclusively to symptoms in the leg. Both, however, may occur simultaneously. The initial symptoms may be described as sharp, dull, continuous, or intermittent. Numbness of the leg may precede or accompany the symptom of pain. Relationship to activities or positions at which symptoms appear may vary, and various positions or activities may relieve the symptoms or vary the character and extent of the site of the symptoms. All of these variations have a mechanical and patho-physiologic explanation. Careful interpretation of the symptoms does not lead merely to accurate diagnosis but also informs the examiner of the extent of herniation, the exact vertebral level of the hernation, and postulates the course of the disease and its prognosis.

The examination, which is relatively simple and can proceed rapidly, merely verifies the impression created by the history. The necessity of many laboratory tests may be eliminated by careful systematic history and examination.

Sciatic pain is rare in an acute strain with facet impingement. Although pressure from the strain is exerted on the disk, the symptoms actually result from an acute synovitis of the compressed facets or from overstretched ligaments. If sciatic pain is present, the complaint is rarely substantiated by *objective* findings of nerve irritation. Most patients with this condition have relatively free trunk flexion but lack the ability to hyperextend or "arch the back" without causing pain. In trunk flexion the facets are separated or disengaged, whereas in extension they are further "jammed" together and the inflamed surfaces are compressed. The complaint of sciatica actually may be interpreted to be pain caused by spasm of the hamstring muscles and may be bilateral. In this situation, irritation of the nerve at its emergence through' the foramen is a mild compression caused by swelling of the synovium constricting the intervertebral foramen. *No* neurologic deficit may result.

In a severe facet impingement the concomitant muscle spasm may be sufficient to compress the disk to the point of herniation. This herniation in the anterior portion of the foramen, coupled with the posterior synovial swelling and facet impingement, further compresses the nerve root.

Nerve root irritation may cause radiation of pain into the hip region, with no more-distal radiation, and be mistakenly diagnosed as hip pathology, but appropriate tests will eliminate the possibility of the hip being involved. Full-free hip-range of motion, a negative reaction to Fabere or Patrick test, full hip abduction range, and free iliopsoas elongation are not found in hip joint disease. Any one of these signs have always been positive indications of possible hip dysfunction.

Mere contact with a normal nerve root is not enough to cause radiation of pain. Pressure on a normal nerve usually does not cause pain (Lindahl). Pressure must be upon a nerve already inflamed and thus hypersensitive. With a nerve already hypersensitive, any mechanical irritation such as movement, loading, or traction upon the nerve can initiate a pain response. When a nerve has been made hypersensitive from contact by a herniated disk, even normal movements, considered physiological, can initiate pain.

Traction upon a nerve is not necessary to cause pain. Pressure alone upon an irritable nerve can cause pain; therefore, merely standing or sitting, which increases intradiscal pressure and causes further disk bulging, can aggravate radiating pain (Fig. 51). When numbness and weakness replaces or supplements pain, it indicates more massive, more intense, and more prolonged pressure on the nerve. The area of numbness and the location of the weakness relates to the specific nerve *dermatome and myotome* involved (Fig. 56).

Central disk herniation can present a diagnostic problem. This condition exists when the nucleus herniates centrally and presses against the posterior longitudinal ligament and compresses neither nerve root. No leg pain occurs or else there may be only a vague sensation of leg discomfort. Lasegue tests are negative. Straight leg raising may be limited as this movement causes the pelvis to rotate and thus flexes the lumbar spine. In testing for straight leg raising, the pelvis must be prevented from rotating.

If extension of the lumbar spine causes pain in the low back with radiation to the leg, it may indicate herniation of a lower lumbar intervertebral disk (L_{4-5} or L_5-S_1), facet impingement, or herniation of a "higher" lumbar disk (L_{2-3} or L_{3-4}). The history and the clinical determination of the root *level* will help in differentiation.

In a low lumbar disk (L_5-S_1 or L_4-L_5), extension of the low back probably causes sciatic radiculitis by compressing the posterior portion of the annulus and causing further hernation. In herniation of disk material at this level, flexion also causes radicular pain by elongation of the spinal canal and consequent stretching of the nerve root over the protruding disk (Fig. 49).

Pain occurring upon extension of the low back may result from facet encroachment and the resultant synovitis. In this condition, extension is painful and relief is usually gotten from flexing the spine. Here radicular pain is usually absent, neurological signs are not found, and recovery is fairly rapid.

Radiating pain from lumbar extension may occur from herniation of a "high"

92

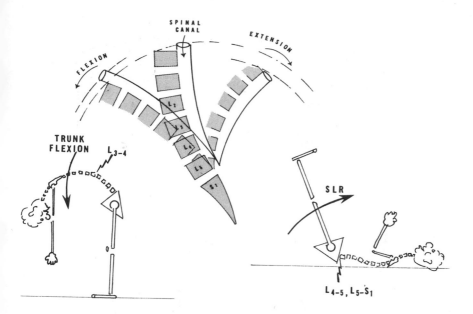

FIGURE 49. Elongation of the spinal canal during flexion. Forward flexion elongates the spinal canal and thus stretches the nerves therein. Movement is greatest in the upper lumbar region. Extension of the low back shortens the canal and the nerves within relax. Straight leg raising, SLR, moves the nerves to a greater degree at the lower lumbar region.

disk (L_{2-3} or L_{3-4}). This tends to occur more in older patients who have moderate disk degeneration. As this degeneration occurs mostly in the lower lumbar disks (L_{4-5} and L_5-S_1), there is excessive motion at the higher levels due to the restriction of the lower vertebrae. As the nerve roots of L_2, L_3, or L_4 are implicated, pain is mediated through the femoral nerve and is felt in the *anterior thigh region* towards the knee region (Fig. 50).

Here the knee jerk is diminished or absent, there is hypalgesia to touch and pin prick over L_2 or L_3 dermatome, and there is weakness of the quadriceps. In time, atrophy of the quadriceps may be noted. Radiation of pain is elicited by stretching the femoral nerve, and this is tested by flexing the knee upon the extended thigh. In the prone position with the thigh extended, stretch pain can be elicited by bringing the heel towards the buttock.

Greater pain occurs on trunk *extension* either when the patient arches backwards or re-arises from a bent position when the pain is caused by facet impingement. Likewise more severe pain occurs from trunk *flexion* in a disk herniation. In both conditions straight leg raising may register "positive" insofar as any movement of the pelvis in such instances causes pain and thus is restricted. Time and observation of the progression of the illness may be necessary to pinpoint ultimately the diagnosis. Fortunately, the treatment of both conditions is essentially the same, as will be discussed in the chapter on

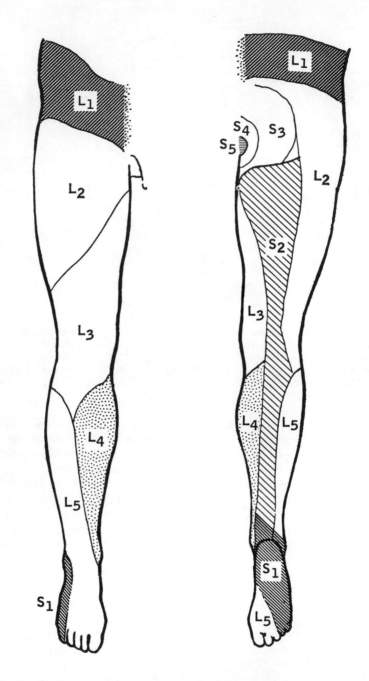

FIGURE 50. Sensory dermatome area map. The areas mapped out are the areas of hypalgesia to pin-scratch testing. There is variation from patient to patient so that the areas at best are general and overlapping.

the treatment of these patients. Little is lost by procrastinating and the patient's welfare will not be jeopardized.

Persistence of scoliosis with limitation of trunk flexion and persistence of pain upon the exercise of straight leg raising unilaterally or bilaterally, in spite of intensive conservative treatment, favors the diagnosis of central disk herniation rather than facet impingement. In "facet" synovitis, the articulations ultimately disengage, straight leg raising becomes possible even to full elevation, the scoliosis gradually decreases, trunk flexion increases in range and smoothness, and mere hyperextension of the low back may remain limited and painful.

The presence of pain running down the leg elicited by coughing or sneezing is strongly suggestive of disk herniation, but this is *not conclusive*. Coughing, especially if violent, can aggravate any type of backache. To accomplish its intended purpose, coughing must stimulate a sudden increase of intrapleural and intra-abdominal pressure. When there is a combination of this violent internal pressure increase and the simultaneous external muscular contraction, all the components contributing to low back discomfort are effected.

Although pain noted in the low back following the act of coughing is not diagnostic of disk herniation, the presence of pain running along the length of the leg after a simulated act of coughing is very suggestive of such interpretation.

Such pain in the leg can be frequently caused or aggravated by forceful flexion of the neck. In the straight leg raising test, after the legs have reached a degree of elevation sufficient to cause pain, flexion of the neck at this point will intensify the sciatic pain. Neck flexion causes traction movement to occur in the dura and arachnoid, and, with an inflamed nerve within the foramen, the traction increases the irritation. The straight leg raising exercise causes movement of the lower nerve-roots, and neck flexion increases the movement of the nerve roots.

The case history frequently relates causation, aggravation, or relief of pain to the effects of gravity. The patient is pain free lying down but feels pain immediately or after a brief period of standing. Sitting is often more painful than standing, and the patient admits he "must stand or walk" to relieve the pain he incurred during sitting.

The hydrodynamics of the lumbar disk can explain this phenomenon. The intradiscal pressure (pressure *within* the nucleus) in a supine person is 30 per cent less than the pressure standing and 50 per cent less than during sitting. The pressure within a lumbar disk is thus greatest during sitting, significantly less in standing, and least when reclining. These findings explain the relief of symptoms when a patient assumes complete bed rest (Fig. 51).

Bending forward from the standing or sitting position with a weight held in the hands, arms held slightly forward, increases the intradiscal pressure. Twisting or turning the trunk applies torque stress to the disks which also increases the intradiscal pressures. This accounts for the frequent story of the patient that he "felt sudden pain in the low back (and leg) on bending forward in a twisted direction to lift an object from the floor." The maneuver is traumatic though the object lifted may be light or insignificant (Fig. 52).

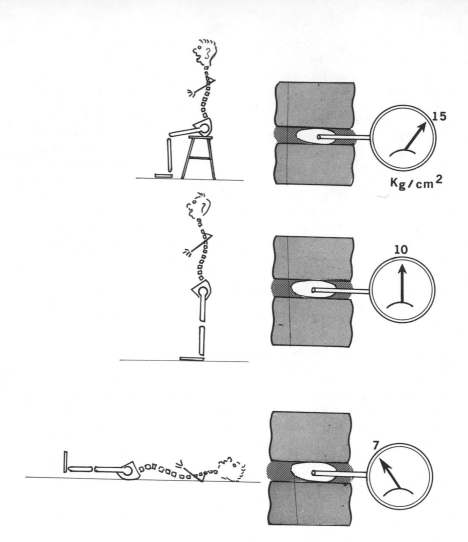

FIGURE 51. Variations in the intradiscal pressure. There is pressure within the nucleus even in the reclining position; it is increased upon standing and is even greater on sitting. Leaning forward with a weight in the hands held forward further increases the pressure within the disk.

Increased abdominal support with pressure upon the abdominal wall, such as wearing a girdle, brace, or lumbosacral corset, decreases the intradiscal pressure. This has been verified experimentally and explains, in part, the rationale of prescribing a girdle or corset for the relief of low back and sciatic pain.

The history of sciatica related by the patient is an expose of *where, when,* and *how* the nerve root is irritated. The physical examination is essentially a confirmatory step in reaching a diagnosis.

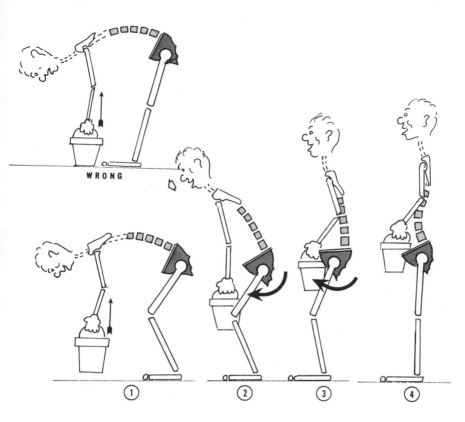

FIGURE 52. Proper technique of lifting. The wrong way of lifting places excessive strain upon the back, thigh muscles, and low back. Properly, the knees should be bent, the object to be lifted kept close to the body (between the feet if possible) (1), the pelvis should be tucked under (2), and when the pelvis is completely "tilted" and the body erect (3), the legs are extended (4).

As in the examination of the patient with low back pain caused by a mechanical defect, the standing posture and its deviation from the normal curves must be evaluated in the case of suspected disk herniation. Excessive lordosis implies merely an increase in the lumbosacral angle insofar as *spasm* rarely causes an increase in sway. Lumbar spasm usually causes a *flattening* of the lordotic curve as well as effecting a lateral scoliosis. Clinically, this flattening is evident in that the erect patient appears to be standing slightly bent forward in the lumbar region. It is of interest to note that the x-ray of the lumbar spine interpreted as showing spasm is so interpreted because the lumbar curve is straightened out (Fig. 53), and consequently the lumbar lordosis obliterated.

Scoliosis is usually present in lumbar disk herniation. The lateral "shunt" of the lumbar spine is most frequently to the side of the nerve root irritation. This is not a constant factor, and probably is offered too frequently as a diagnostic sign in determining which side of the disk is herniated. The segmental spasm

97

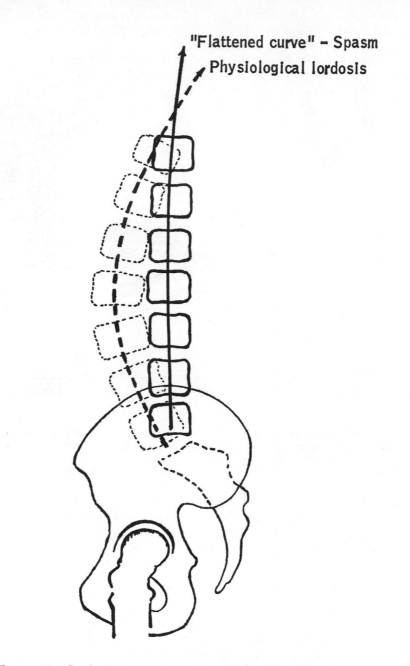

"Flattened curve" – Spasm

Physiological lordosis

FIGURE 53. Lumbar spasm with resultant "flattening." The spasm resulting from nerve root irritation causes a protective spasm. This spasm, rather than increasing the lordosis, results in straightening the lumbar curve. Further forward flexion of the lumbar curve is prevented by this spasm.

ca...sing acute scoliosis is undoubtedly the result of a splinting action caused by nerve-root recurrent nerve irritation, and the spasm involves a segment of several vertebrae (Fig. 54).

Spasm is detected during the examination when the patient attempts to bend at the waist, with no consequent reversal of the lordosis. This protective spasm preventing flexion is largely segmental and unilateral and will intensify the scoliosis during the course of flexion.

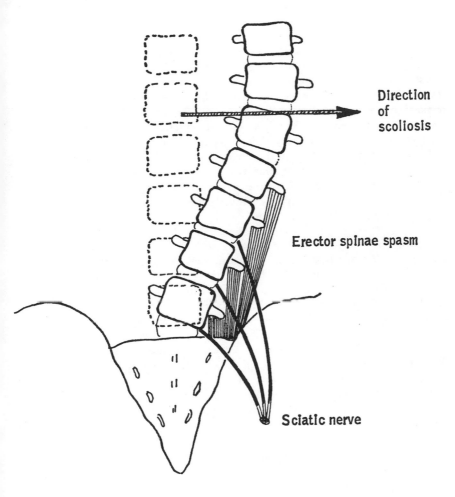

Direction of scoliosis

Erector spinae spasm

Sciatic nerve

FIGURE 54. Mechanism of acute protective scoliosis. Irritation of the nerve root at its emergence through the intervertebral foramen causes reflex spasm, usually on the same side as the site of irritation. By its segmental distribution, only a small portion of the paraspinous muscles is involved and thus a segmental lateral curve of the spine results.

Limited trunk flexion because of spasm acting as a protective mechanism can be understood when it is realized that trunk flexion normally causes traction on the dural sac. Flexion of the trunk causes an upward movement of the spinal nerves. This movement is most marked at the L_1-L_2 level and movement of the nerves decreases caudally so that trunk flexion causes no significant movement of the nerve root at the L_5 level and actually very little movement, if any, at the L_4 level.

Limitation of lateral movement of the lumbar spine is not useful in diagnosis. Lateral movement is insignificant in the normal kinetic function of the lumbar spine because of the planes and relationship of the facets. Spasm which originates as a protective device must prevent physiologic movement and in turn must prevent flexion and extension. The restriction of *lateral* flexibility from spasm is part of the total restriction of all spinal movements.

Significant restriction of lumbar flexion which might serve diagnostic purposes must be viewed in respect to the degree of limitation imposed upon the reversal action of the lordotic curve during attempted trunk flexion. No numeral expression of flexion limitation can be so formulated that it will reserve reversal acceptance. Merely an estimate described as either full, slight, incomplete, or partial reversal of lordosis on flexion can be made and recorded.

The *straight leg raising test* is a delicate and accurate neurologic test. The straight leg raising test (from this point to be designated the *SLR*) is currently used interchangeably with the terms *positive* or *negative* Lasegue sign. The SLR, when done carefully, and properly interpreted, is one of the few tests that offer objective diagnostic signs.

The SLR is not in actuality the Lasegue sign. In the SLR, the leg is flexed at the hip with the knee held in full extension. The ankle, during the exercise, remains in a relaxed position. Forst was the first to describe this test. The test described by Lasegue was that of flexion of the hip to 90 degrees, followed by extension of the lower leg in line with the thigh. The term *Lasegue* has now clinical acceptance as being synonymous with SLR. If, however, either test is interpreted correctly, the designation employed is of no importance.

During SLR the first 15 to 30 degrees of elevation causes no movement of the nerve roots at the foraminal level. But when the leg has reached an angle of 30 degrees, there is traction on the sciatic nerve followed by a downward movement of the roots in their foramina. The greatest degree of movement occurs in the L_5 root, some slight movement at L_4, and essentially no movement at L_2 or L_3. The greatest distance of any root movement, a distance of two to five millimeters (2-5 mm.), occurs when the SLR has brought the leg to an angle of 60 to 80 degrees (Fig. 55).

The clinical interpretation urged by these facts is that owing to the greatest downward movement occurring at the L_5 level, a disk herniation at this level will have a strongly felt positive reaction from the SLR. As there is a decreasing amount of reaction at the higher nerve root levels, a disk herniation at the level of L_3 or even L_4 may not produce a positive SLR. A positive SLR is of greatest value in helping to locate a disk herniation at the L_5-S_1 and L_{4-5} level, but its absence does not argue against a disk herniation existing at a higher interspace.

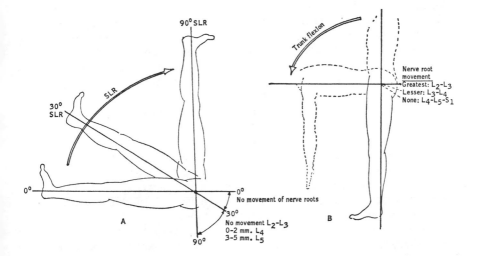

FIGURE 55. A, The degree of nerve root movement that occurs at the intervertebral foramen in the SLR test. No movement occurs at any vertebral level in the first 30 degrees of SLR. At 60 to 80 degrees of SLR, maximum movement of nerve roots occurs with 3 to 5 mm. of the nerve at L_5-S_1 to no movement at L_2-L_3. B, Opposite traction movement in trunk flexing as compared to SLR in that greatest movement occurs at L_2-L_3 in trunk flexion and no root movement at L_5-S_1 level.

In view of the movement noted at the lower intervertebral level from SLR and conversely (at the L_5 level) the very slight movement occurring from trunk flexion, it follows that there is greater specificity of the SLR test in lower disk herniations and greater specificity of trunk flexion at higher nerve-root levels. There is, it must be recalled, an insignificant degree of nerve-root movement at L_5 from trunk flexion; thus simple trunk flexion in the presence of a low (L_5-S_1) disk herniation may cause no sciatic-like pain. Spasm occurring in the lower region of the back is a splinting mechanism initiated by irritation of recurrent spinal-nerve irritation. Its function is apparently not merely to prevent trunk flexion as much as to prevent nerve-root movement in the foraminal space.

The SLR of one leg causes the lower lumbar roots on the opposite side to descend caudally and thus causes these contralateral nerves to emerge from their foramen and approach the anterior wall or the disk area. In the ipsilateral SLR, as the greatest movement occurs at the lowest segmental level so the greatest contralateral movement also exists at the lower nerve roots.

Another test that may be added to the SLR series is that of forcefully dorsiflexing the foot at the ankle, once the pain-free extent of SLR has been reached. Frequently this maneuver of ankle flexion will elicit pain in the area of the sciatic nerve distribution when the mere SLR test of itself is at best equivocal. This modification is of greatest value when the defective condition is present unilaterally and is discovered only to one side and when the patient's leg in the SLR reaches a degree less than the normal.

A different manner of performing the SLR test that has proved of sufficient value to merit discussion has been that of performing the test while the patient is sitting. With legs dangling, the patient is seated on the edge of the table, and faces the examiner. The test then is merely performed by extending the patient's legs below the knee one at a time. The examiner should note the results objectively and subjectively.

This apparently trivial modification of the test described by Lasegue in respect to the supine position has several benefits. In the supine position, raising a straight leg manually can be difficult because the patient may squirm and shift his pelvis, thus making the leg abduct and rotate. Furthermore the apprehension of the patient to ward off anticipated pain may cause SLR to render positive reaction far sooner than the objective facts warrant. In the supine position the back may be in a flexed or an extended position which may influence the test and cause difficulty in its proper interpretation.

In the sitting position, however, the patient faces the examiner and feels more secure and at ease. The examiner is able to determine immediately the slightest attempt on the part of the patient to withdraw by leaning back from the pain induced by the straight leg raising. Indication that the pain level has been reached may be given by the facial grimace of the patient or by his "general bracing" against further leg-elevation. Furthermore, it is no easier to note and record the precise degree of elevation (viz., 45°, 65°, etc.) from the test taken in the supine position. Neither method can be said to be more accurate or significant than the other.

The results of the SLR should be expressed in the terms of positive or negative. The test is essentially a qualitative test rather than a quantitative test. SLR is an objective and an accurate test when the results are correctly determined as being "positive." The presence of a crossed sciatic pain showing up on contralateral SLR is equally objective and informative. It is obvious that a crossed sciatica response is rarely elicited with a negative ipsilateral SLR.

In patients suspected of falsifying or magnifying their symptoms the method of doing the SLR test with the subject seated has a disarming and distracting effect on the patient. The test can be performed with complete unawareness on the part of the patient. The leg can be slowly elevated, under the guise of checking the pulses at the ankle, "feeling the skin," or looking at the veins. A SLR can frequently be performed while the patient is assisted in removing his shoes or stockings.

Many a "positive" SLR may elicit severe pain and resistance at 45 degrees of elevation. But the doctor may find that he can raise the patients' leg to a 90 degree angle under the guise of "checking the circulation," or testing for a flat-footed condition, but when a patient responds to the doctor's examination by leaning backwards, by grimacing when one leg and not the other is raised, he is offering a reaction far more significant than those expressing a "positive Lasegue at 65 degrees on the right leg and 70 degrees on the left."

Neurologic Examination and Interpretation

After the presence of sciatic nerve irritation has been established and its segmental level indicated in the history, the neurologic examination now confirms the root level. Limited trunk flexibility with or without scoliosis implicates the lumbar level as the gross site of trouble. A positive SLR heightens the probability of a lower segment rather than a higher level being involved (S_1 rather than L_3, for instance). The patient's statement and description of the area of pain referral or area of altered sensation gives an estimated zone for dermatome referral and indicates the extent of the nerve root under pressure.

The neurologic examination can now objectively confirm the site of nerve involvement earlier implied in the history. Again when the patient sits and faces the examiner, he permits a careful and complete examination with a minimum of movement involved. The details of the neurologic examination will be discussed only as they pertain to lumbar disk herniation. Neuropathy from disk herniation is equivalent to the studies of peripheral spinal nerve dysfunction. Any suspicion of upper motor deficit or cord involvement relegates further studies to the specialty of the neurologist or the neurosurgeon. The essence of the present neurologic examination is summarized in Fig. 56.

During the first phase of the examination previously described in which the standing posture was examined, the opportunity to examine the integrity of the S_1 myotome presented itself. Having the patient stand on one foot and arise up and down on his toes tests the strength and endurance of the calf muscles, the gastrocnemius-soleus group. The gastrocnemius-soleus muscle group is supplied by the S_1 myotome which emerges in the interspace between L_5 and the first sacral vertebra S_1.

The gastrocnemius is a powerful muscle, capable of lifting the patient's full body weight with additional weight superimposed. It is practically impossible for the examiner to test this muscle manually or to determine its endurance unless the muscle is markedly paretic. When a patient in upright position arises on the toes of one foot at a time, the full body weight of the patient will reveal weakness relatively early and will reveal slight degrees of weakness not possible by manual testing.

Minor impairment of the S_1 myotome may cause a fatigability, rather than significant weakness readily determined from one resisted active contraction. The presence of fatigability is a more delicate demonstration of minimal impairment and is one found relatively early in root compression. Determination of as powerful a muscle as the gastrocnemius by resistance to normal manipulation would obviously be difficult, if not impossible.

Susceptibility to fatigue can be established and ascertained by having the patient arise up and down on one foot repeatedly. Fatigue, so determined, can be recorded in an objective quantitative manner for later comparative tests.

Testing the anterior tibialis muscle, the ankle dorsiflexors, when the patient is standing or walking on his heels, is not a very delicate test. The L_4-L_5 myotomes are more accurately tested with the patient seated, legs dangling from the table. If there is sufficient weakness of the anticus muscle the patient may describe a "drop foot" gait, the presence of which can be verified by observa-

Nerve Root	Inter-vert. Space	Subjective Pain Radiation	Sensory Area	Bladder Bowel Dysfunction	SLR	AJ	KJ	Motor Dysfunction (Myotome)
L₃	L₂-L₃	Back to buttocks to posterior thigh to anterior knee region	Hypalgesia in knee region	+/−	Usually −	+	+	Quadriceps Weakness
L₄	L₃-L₄	Back to buttocks to posterior thigh to inner calf region	Hypalgesia inner aspect of lower leg	+/−	Usually − May be +	+	−	Quadriceps and possible anticus weakness
L₅	L₄-L₅	Back to buttocks to —(etc.)— dorsum of foot and big toe	Hypalgesia in dorsum foot and big toe	+/−	++	+	+	Weakness of anterior tibialis, big toe extensor, gluteus medius
S₁	L₅-S₁	Back to buttocks to —(etc.)— sole of foot and heel	Hypalgesia in heel or lateral foot	+/−	+++	−	+	Weakness of gastrocnemius, hamstring, gluteus maximus
				*	**	***		****

FIGURE 56. Schematic dermatome and myotome level of nerve root impingement.

 * Bladder and bowel dysfunction can occur at any level.
 ** Related to extent of nerve root movement at each level.
 *** AJ is absent only at L₅-S₁; KJ at L₃-L₄ (see text).
 **** Only the more obvious and functional muscles are listed. (This is not a complete list of muscles innervated.)

tion of the patient's walking pattern. For finer evaluation of anterior tibialis weakness, having the patient dorsiflex his ankle against resistance for strength or maintain the full dorsiflexion against maintained pressure for endurance will elicit L_5 myotome impairment.

The strength of the hamstring group in their knee flexing action is best tested while the patient is seated and bends his knee to bring his lower leg under the table. In this position, movement done against resistance is better than the standard method of testing with the patient lying in the prone position. In the prone attitude there is marked tendency to arch the back which is not evident when the patient is sitting. Avoidance of too much reclining, turning, sitting, and rolling over is desirable for a patient with a low back pain or herniated lumbar disk. The hamstring muscle group is innervated by S_1 primarily and confirms weakness already noted in the gastrocnemius-soleus (S_1) and the big toe extensor (S_1).

To test the higher nerve roots (L_3-L_4) the strength of the quadriceps femoris group is tested. This muscle group extends the leg at the knee. As the quadriceps muscle is very powerful, it may be necessary to have the person do repeated one-legged deep knee bends to determine fatigue as well as weakness. In more marked weakness the patient, while in the sitting position, may be unable to maintain full extension of the leg at the knee against slight manual pressure. The quadriceps strength test may be invalidated in the presence of a painful SLR when the testing is done with the patient seated. If sciatic neuritis or tight hamstrings is suspected of restricting knee extension, the quadriceps may be tested with the patient supine.

It is seriously recommended that the patient be examined in the *upright* position when the strength of the antigravity muscle is tested. The present-day manner of examining the patient draped and lying on an examining table leaves many significant factors unnoticed. Even the examination with the patient in a sitting position is inadequate for thorough evaluation. Where this applies in posture and kinetic function evaluation, so in the same way it must be employed in muscle testing. It is inconceivable that in an attempt to determine deviation from normal, man should not be examined in his normal upright stance and in his antigravity functions.

Further phases of the neurologic examination can also be performed with the patient seated. After the completion of the SLR testing, examination of the deep tendon jerks is made. The reflexes are evaluated with reference to their presence, and comparison is made of relation of one side to the other. The deep tendon reflexes reflect peripheral nerve integrity and therefore are a test of lower motor neuron function. In essence the reflexes are tested to determine the spinal segmental level of any suspected nerve root compression. Depression of one side as compared to the other is of significance because pressure on the nerve root will result in depression of the reflex. Significant pressure on a nerve root may result in total loss of a deep tendon reflex.

The ankle jerk (AJ) is dependent on an intact S_1 motor root. A depressed knee jerk (KJ) implicates pressure on the L_4 root. Active symmetrical knee and ankle jerks are expected when there is nerve root compression at L_5 as this nerve root does not innervate a tendon reflex. Pressure on the nerve root

105

at this level (L_5) requires sensory and motor testing to establish the diagnosis.

Absence of *bilateral* deep tendon reflexes at one level is possible in a central disk herniation at a segmental level when both left and right nerve roots are encroached upon. Although neither motor nor sensory deficit may exist with areflexia, some nerve impairment exists, and other signs of lumbar-disk herniation should exist, such as bilateral positive SLR reactions, lumbar spine spasm, scoliosis, and subjective unilateral or bilateral sciatica.

The sensory examination follows in the neurologic appraisal. A pin is "run down" (that is, applied with a light scratching maneuver rather than by "sticking") the inner side of each leg into the foot area, then down the lateral aspect of the legs, the bilateral heel areas, lateral aspects of the foot, and the dorsum of the big toes. This method aids the patient to ascertain differences more easily as the dermatome maps overlap and the scratch does not demand a distinct border of any area. These areas have been depicted in Fig. 50. Suffice to say that the *difference* of sensation of the right compared to left is the objective of the test—not merely the ability of the patient "to feel the pin scratch." Nerve root compression results in impaired sensation of the specific dermatome area, varying from hypalgesia to complete anaesthesia. Hyperesthesia on the basis of nerve irritation is rarely found in nerve root involvement due to disk protrusion, although it is theoretically possible to have irritation hyperesthesia.

Confirmatory Tests

A working diagnosis is reached by the history and physical examination. There are confirmatory x-ray evidence and laboratory tests that deserve mention, although their thorough discussion and evaluation are beyond the scope of this presentation. The doctor should at least have an idea when to request such tests and how much can be gained from them. The interpretation of the specific tests, such as x-ray, electromyogram, and myelogram, is a function of the specialist in that field, but the doctor who has requested the report should be qualified to interpret the findings reported.

The value of confirmatory tests is limited but is specific. No individual test of its own is completely diagnostic. As in any field of medicine, laboratory tests should be considered as supplementary and confirmatory to the history and physical examination. Some of these tests will not be necessary, and it is the decision of the doctor to accept or reject certain tests. The doctor should certainly be able to explain their value to the patient as well as intelligently to discuss their results with the consultant.

X-ray studies by routine films are of surprisingly little value in the diagnosis of herniated lumbar disks. Finding "normal disk spaces" does not exclude the presence of disk herniation. X-rays do not in themselves localize the level of disk herniation causing clinical symptoms. Radiologic evidence of a "narrow disk space" merely indicates that the disk material has been extruded or is to some degree degenerated. When the intradiskal pressure that normally maintains separation of the vertebrae permits a narrowing of the intervertebral disk space, it is obviously deficient and this deficiency implies the presence of rupture or degeneration, but the x-ray will not differentiate between these two entities.

When a narrowed intervertebral disk space is roentgenologically found with "marginal sclerosis" of the vertebral bodies and some degree of osteophyte formation or spur (so-called evidence of *osteoarthritis*) the only conclusion that can be drawn at the time is that there is degeneration of the disk in addition to some efforts made by nature to effect repair. The finding of hypertrophic spurs by x-ray does not of itself incriminate the spurs as the cause of nerve root impingement. On the other hand, evidence of disk degeneration with marginal sclerosis and osteophyte formation indicates long-existing disk degeneration undergoing repair, but does not eliminate the possibility of an acute herniation of that particular disk.

X-rays are frequently taken for psychological reasons; the patient may have the feeling that x-rays must be taken or that without them the examination is not complete. This practice, which gives assurance to the patient, is also beneficial to the doctor. In today's medical care, the medicolegal claims of "neglect" must also always be kept in mind, and x-ray pictures, necessary or not, become imperative from a medicolegal standpoint.

Electromyography objectively confirms motor nerve-root involvement and localizes the root segment involved. The EMG is a localizing diagnostic tool and a test that objectively verifies motor involvement when the clinical picture is non-specific. An EMG is a qualitative, not a quantitative test. It merely tells which nerve or nerves are impaired but does not specify the degree of impairment, and in the early course of the illness is not a prognosticating instrument.

The EMG, however, is an objective test since the EMG results can be recorded. Conversion hysterical patterns can be differentiated from organic nerve damage. Differentiation of weakness resulting from pain which decreases the voluntary effort is easily differentiated by EMG from weakness caused by nerve pathology. An EMG test, however, is of no value during the first three weeks immediately following nerve pressure as the presence of nerve demyelinization necessary for giving a positive EMG test is not present for 21 days. Long after disk pressure on a nerve has subsided and function is returning clinically, the EMG will still continue to show fibrillation of demyelinization so that it cannot be used to specify exactly when nerve pressure is released.

No more than confirmation of a clinical impression, therefore, is to be demanded or expected of electromyography.

Myelography, or Pantopaque study, is not usually necessary to make the diagnosis of radiculopathy. The test is difficult, not without hazard, and not without discomfort to the patient. Myelography can be considered necessary when certain conditions have been verified. First it is employed when the decision has been made to treat the herniated disk surgically, thus implying that further conservative therapy is no longer considered profitable. The myelogram now specifically localizes the lesion and confirms the probability of finding a herniated disk during the operation. Secondly, a myelogram ascertains preoperatively the presence of one or two disk herniations. Thirdly, it aids in the differential diagnosis of herniated lumbar disk versus caudal equinal tumor when the latter possibility is entertained clinically. Fourthly, it affirms the recurrence of disk herniation when symptoms suggest this recurrence after the patient has had previous disk surgery. Lastly, the rare incidence of persistent low back pain with trunk limitation without subjective or objective nerve root irritation clinically evident may be attributed to a central disk herniation by myelography.

Pathology is found upon operation in an estimated 85 per cent of patients who had a positive Lasegue test and some neurological deficit such as reflex changes, sensory loss, or motor deficit preoperatively. If the myelogram also is abnormal the probability of finding an offending herniated disk is even greater (90 per cent).

Even with a "negative" myelogram, surgery is indicated when there are sufficient neurological findings in the presence of a consistent history. Here the decision must be based on the intensity and duration of the pain, the extent of the neurological deficit, and its failure to respond to conservative treatment after a sufficiently long trial period.

Doctors differ somewhat in what they interpret as a "positive" myelogram. This dye test is considered "positive" if the dural sac is deformed at the suspected disk level, the root is displaced from its normal position as compared to the normal side, and the root sleeve does not fill with the contrast dye material.

Under no circumstances need a myelogram be performed as a routine laboratory procedure when no serious doubt regarding diagnosis exists. This is also true where conservative treatment has *not* been tried, when surgery is *not* imminent, or when, even in the advent of finding a defect consistent with disk herniation in the myelogram, surgery for other reasons will *not* be considered in the treatment.

Diskography has become more popular in an attempt to "specifically localize the offending disk" and to establish that the "disk protrusion is the cause of the patient's symptoms." Injection of dye into the suspected disk will reveal that the nucleus has degenerated and escaped its boundaries into the annular tears. The increase of pressure from the injected dye should reproduce the patient's symptoms, verifying the "exact level of the offending disk."

The diskogram can visualize that the disk is degenerated and even "ruptured" but the reproduction of the symptoms is difficult to evaluate. Injection into disks at two or more levels may evoke the symptoms, but the patient is unable to differentiate which location produces the symptoms.

Furthermore, finding an abnormal diskogram does not eliminate the presence of other pathology such as an extradural tumor, spondylosis, or arachnoiditis as the cause of the symptoms and findings. Diskography has not yet adequately replaced the objectivity of proper neurological examination and properly interpreted myelograms.

Conservative Treatment

Because conservative *treatment* of the patient with a herniated lumbar disk

108

is so often necessary and useful, it is important at this juncture to consider the procedure thoroughly.

Elimination of Gravity. One of the first factors to be accounted for is gravity, a strong compression force acting on the disk; therefore the elimination of the stress of gravity is the first requirement in the treatment. Eliminating gravity means bed rest in every aspect that the term "bed rest" denotes. *Bed rest must be complete, continuous, correct, and sufficiently prolonged.*

Such bed rest must demand a firm bed. Firmness actually demands the presence of a board under the mattress. The board must be as long and as wide as the mattress and must be at least 3/4 to 1 inch thick. The reason for this specified thickness is that a thinner board will sag when supporting the weight of a person lying in the center of the bed. Even ¼-inch board supported at its ends will sag.

Any mattress from 4 to 6 inches in thickness placed on the board will suffice. The mattress by its compressibility merely prevents pressure points on bony prominences of the body and it is to be repeated no mattress, no matter how constructed, without a thick supporting board, will prevent central sagging.

The board should preferably be a "split" board; i.e., cut in three sections and held together by hinges. This type of board permits placing the patient in a semi-Fowler position, which is the desirable position for prolonged bed rest. The semi-Fowler position as applied here indicates a semi-sitting posture with slight flexion of the hips and knees. (The true original "Fowler position" consisted merely in the elevation of the head of the bed to insure drainage of the abdominal cavity by gravity; hence, the current use of the term *Fowler* is actually a misnomer.) The slightly flexed position by flattening the lumbar spine and flexing the hips eliminates hip-flexor stretch. The bent knee position relieves the tension from the hamstrings exerted on the pelvis. In this position the patient is better able to withstand the duration of the bed rest that is required for "healing" of disk bulging or herniation.

In the hospital, this flexed semi-Fowler position is easily maintained and because of the modern hospital bed, the position of the patient can easily be adjusted. At home the split board as described is readily available and, by the use of cushions or pillows, the same position as in the hospital bed can be maintained. There is no reason, however, for *not* permitting a flat bed if the patient can be comfortable and, in this flat position, will remain at bed rest.

Bathroom privileges must be curtailed. In the male patient, bladder function presents no problem; the urinal, or a wide-mouth bottle, will suffice. For the female patient, the bedpan poses more difficulty owing to its awkwardness and the necessity for assistance in using it. For bowel function, the bedpan presents the same difficulty for both sexes because of inconvenience and discomfort inherent in its use.

Patients with a herniated lumbar disk frequently have a pain-initiated reflex ileus or experience constipation caused by the prescribed medication. These factors combined with the pain from straining or from the effort made in even assuming the position on a bedpan in bed may intensify not only the constipation but may also aggravate the disk herniation. For these reasons, controlled bathroom privileges may sometimes be more sensible than insistence upon use of a bedpan.

Bathroom privileges must never be granted if the bed is too high for easy descent and the distance to the bathroom too long. The bed must be sufficiently low to permit the patient to place his feet on the floor immediately upon reaching the sitting position. This poses a nursing problem because an attendant is inconvenienced in making a low bed and must nurse the patient on that level. Whatever the hardship to the nursing personnel, for the patient's sake and comfort, this low bed is a necessity if bathroom privileges are to be considered

For the short-distance walk to the bathroom the use of crutches will minimize the weight-bearing factors. The use of a bedside commode is worthy of consideration, but if the use of the bedpan is deemed necessary, this can be facilitated by having an overhead trapeze or "monkey bar" from which the patient may elevate and suspend himself while the pan is placed and removed.

The proper way for the patient with a backache to get out of bed merits discussion. The method of arising from the supine position should be taught the patient. The proper sequence of getting out of bed is to turn on one's side, draw the knees up to a semi-flexed position, push down on the bed with the upper-most arm and simultaneously support the partially elevated body on the dependent elbow. Having gained this position, the patient can now sit up by simply straightening the bent, dependent arm. While the arm is pushing the body away from the bed to the erect sitting position, the flexed hips and knee are slowly swung over the edge of the bed. Performing these progressive stages, the body is moved as a unit with the lumbar spine remaining in a flexed position and the hips and knees remaining flexed. No strain on the low back results, and the patient moves with confidence and a minimum of discomfort.

Bed Exercise. Bed exercises are to be begun immediately, but are to be carefully prescribed and judiciously increased. The major purpose of early exercise is to maintain limberness and benefit general circulation. Merely lying immobile in a prone position causes unnecessary discomfort and, if prolonged, ultimately causes myostatic contractures and pressure points on the body. Disuse atrophy begins early as does general debility. Although bed rest is usually not so prolonged in the treatment of disk disease, the reconditioning of the patient after recovery, or postoperatively in the patient who ultimately requires surgery, is greatly aided by early exercises.

The first exercise is the movement of "knee to chest" done gently and rhythmically. Brief periods of exercising done frequently rather than prolonged bouts of exercising are desirable. After each leg separately is flexed to the chest, the action of both "knees to chest" is added. No straining should result from doing these exercises, and no significant pain should occur during or after the exercise. Muscle setting exercises (isometric contractions) of the muscles of the legs and arms aid in heightening the circulation, muscle relaxation, and in the prevention of disuse atrophy.

Medication. Relaxation of muscle spasm is secondary only to the elimination of gravity in treating the disk herniation syndrome. No drug on the market at this time is totally effective in relaxing muscle spasm which is initiated by nerve irritation and pain. The ideal drug should have a muscle relaxing effect, a tranquilizing effect to decrease psychic tension, and a mild sedative effect to increase the pain-threshold and encourage the patient to await natural healing in a relaxed manner. Such drugs may have to be given orally or hypodermically as dictated by the patient's condition and should be devoid of as many side reactions as possible. Personal experience of the doctor is the best evaluation of the medicine's efficacy and of the necessary dosage.

Traction. In medical as well as lay parlance, the use of traction has gained the reputation of being the specific treatment for ruptured disks. There are as many techniques for applying traction as the many theories of what traction does. The supposition, or premise, that traction "separates the lumbar vertebrae and permits the disk to return in its container" is without basis and is an untenable conclusion. The value of traction is probably twofold; properly applied traction (1) decreases the lumbar lordosis and (2) decreases the muscle spasm. The flattening of the lumbar lordosis opens the posterior aspect of the functional unit and thus increases the intervertebral foraminal aperture. Decrease of muscle spasm probably results as much from the enforced bed rest and medication as from any single factor of traction. It is possible that the maintained elongation effect on the muscles may fatigue the hypertonus and induce relaxation by fatigue of the muscle tone, but the truth of this theory has yet to be proved.

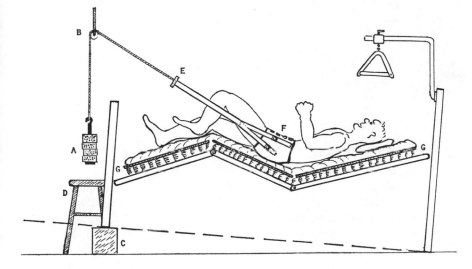

FIGURE 57. Pelvic traction with the patient in a "semi-Fowler position." The patient is wearing a pelvic band with the pull acting so as to flex the lumbar spine.

A, Weights applying the traction, usually 20 lbs.

B, Overhead pulley so placed that the pull tilts or lifts the pelvis.

C, Ten-inch block to elevate foot of bed.

D, Stool to support the weights when patient temporarily disengages them.

E, Spreader bar to separate the lateral straps pulling on the pelvic band around patient's pelvis.

F, Pelvic band with buckles to permit easy detachment by patient.

G, Split board between mattress and box springs to prevent sagging.

111

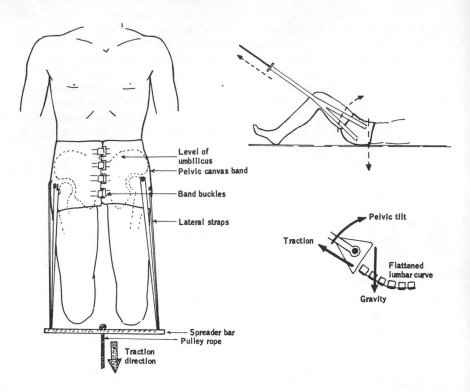

Level of
umbilicus
Pelvic canvas band

Band buckles

Lateral straps

Pelvic tilt

Traction

Flattened
lumbar curve

Gravity

Spreader bar
Pulley rope

Traction
direction

FIGURE 58.   Equipment for pelvic traction. Drawing at left depicts method of attaching pelvic traction equipment. The lateral straps are placed to permit leg movements and exercises in bed. Drawing at the right discloses the resultant pelvic rotation gained by this method of applying traction.

Traction applied by means of bilateral Buck's traction affixed by adhesive attachments to each lower leg is undesirable. The force of traction applied in this manner is dissipated at the knee and hip joints and results in arching the back rather than in decreasing the lordosis. The patient so connected to his traction equipment is restricted to the fully elongated position and is prevented from arising unless the traction is disconnected. This is a time-consuming procedure. Bathroom privileges are precluded and nursing care becomes mandatory. Not the least significant and undesirable aspect of Buck's traction is the difficulty of performing at periodic intervals an accurate and thorough neurologic examination on a patient swathed in bandages.

Pelvic traction is the most physiologic, most comfortable, and the easiest method of traction to apply and maintain (Fig. 57). A snug pelvic band from which the traction is exerted fits above and on the iliac crest of the pelvis (Fig. 58). Lateral bands attached to the pelvic band exert equal pull on the

112

left and right side and must be placed laterally and posteriorly to "lift" the pelvis while they have the added advantage of simultaneously applying traction. The lateral bands must be separated sufficiently to permit movement of the legs between the parallel straps. Separation of these straps, is maintained by a spreader bar.

The pull exerted on the pelvic band via the lateral bands must draw at an angle that elevates the pelvis. Concurrent with the traction elevation of the pelvis, the downward pull of the body weight gives a resultant rotation or "tilt" to the pelvis (Fig. 58). The resultant of these two forces composed of one force in the direction of traction straps and the downward force of the body weight pivoting around a center body point is a single force in a circular direction resulting in rotation and traction.

The foot of the bed should be higher than the head to permit the sliding effect of the patient towards the head of the bed. This will neutralize the traction pulling in the direction of the foot of the bed. Such bed elevation does not cause an uncomfortable dependency of the patient's head.

Conservative treatment of the lumbar disk herniation can thus be summarized as (1) elimination of gravity by bed rest, (2) gentle bed exercises to prevent circulatory stasis, disuse atrophy, and pressure point discomfort, (3) medication to decrease pain, decrease spasm, and tranquillize or sedate the patient, and (4) traction to assist in overcoming lumbar spasm and decrease lumbar lordosis.

It would be difficult to specify the length of time conservative treatment should be maintained. Time required for healing is measured in weeks rather than in days.

Ambulation

After a period of bed rest and traction, usually from two to three weeks' duration, with evidence of subjective and objective improvement, ambulation may be gradually started. The first days of ambulation must be considered as a test to ascertain the strength of the healed annulus in sustaining the added pressure of gravity and movement. If gravity causes a recurrence of disk bulging, there will be recurrence of previous symptoms or a significant increase in the symptoms that had decreased during the period of bed rest.

Bracing and Corseting. Ambulation at first must be undertaken in brief and frequent periods with a minimum of exertion and movement. Corseting or bracing should be considered for early ambulation and the brace should insure a flat lumbar lordosis. The corset chosen should be long. For the adult, of standard height a 16-inch garment is prescribed. The upper portion of the corset should extend from the lower rib cage and the lower edge should reach the inferior crease of the buttocks. The corset should incorporate inflexible steel stays or ribs that extend the full length of the corset. These stays should be flat, without a significant lumbar curve but merely a slight curving at their very base to conform to the lower contour of the buttocks. *The stays should determine the curvature of the spine. The spine should conform to the contour of the stays in the corset. The stays should not conform to the contour of the spine.* The purpose of the corset is to achieve physiologic curving of the spine. It should be added that a smaller corset does not splint and, in fact, by pressing on the mid-portion of the lumbar spine tends to increase lordosis (Fig. 59).

The mechanism by which the immobilization from a brace or corset physiologically benefits a symptomatic discogenic disease is not fully understood. A brace does not eliminate the stresses of gravity. Bracing does restrict flexi-

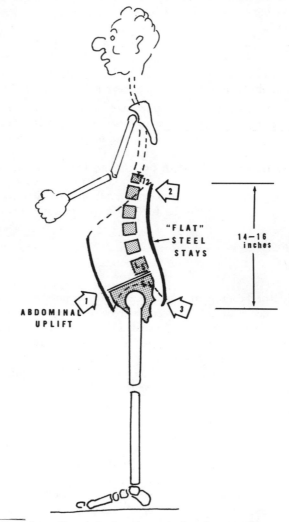

FIGURE 59. Corseting. Proper back support is based on 3 points of contact: Firm uplifting abdominal support (1), back point of contact at thoracolumbar junction (2), and over the sacrum (3). Points 2 and 3 insure that the lumbar curve is "flat," that is the lordosis is decreased.

114

bility, but this cannot be the entire answer. In the presence of spasm, the function of which is to immobilize movement of the spine, the brace replaces the need for the spasm and thus benefits the spine by removing the undesirable effects of spasm. Spasm is considered as undesirable when viewed as an added compressive force on two adjacent vertebrae. The major benefit of bracing must be assumed to be the positioning and maintaining of the spine in proper physiologic curves. For this reason the proper molding of the brace is of the utmost importance.

Proper corseting prevents the relaxed posture previously described as "energy saving" in which the patient leans on his ligamentous structure and thus spares sustained muscular tone. The ligamentous strain and the poor posture that are inherent in this stance are avoided by the support. The muscular effort required to combat the ligamentous supported posture, which is fatiguing and requires concentrated effort, is minimized by bracing (Fig. 60).

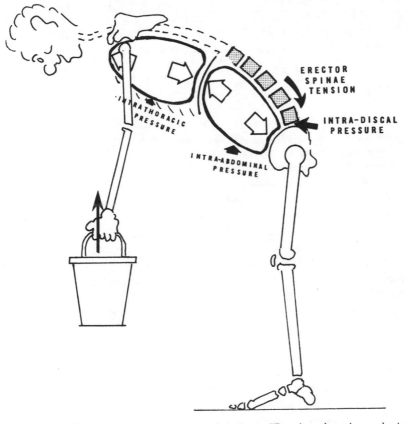

FIGURE 60. Abdominal-thoracic support of spine. The intrathoracic and intra-abdominal pressures created during the act of lifting decrease the pressure exerted by stress forces upon the intervertebral disks. This substantiates the efficacy of a corset, a brace with an abdominal support, and the need for *"strong abdominal muscles to insure a strong back."*

115

Bracing may ultimately serve as a crutch to the patient by accomplishing effortless proper posture that may result in deconditioning. For that reason the corset must be used for a limited time and must be supplemented by proper exercises and constant attention to proper posture. Flexibility must be maintained by means of exercises. It is to be understood that the corset at times can be loosened or briefly removed to permit supine exercises.

At last the time comes for gradual progressive weaning away from the corset. The proper time to begin the weaning varies with each individual case. There is danger in wearing a brace too long, but there must be enough time for sufficiently prolonged support to permit healing. A period from six to eight weeks is the usual minimum time factor.

Reconditioning. Gradually the patient, now pain-free and orthopedically and neurologically "negative," must be reconditioned. All activities are gradually to be resumed, but the need for daily exercises to maintain flexibility and muscle tone must become a ritual. Proper posture and correct kinetic function must be constantly kept in mind. The patient's memory of the once-severe pain and prolonged disability fades in time but is quickly reawakened with the appearance of a slight twinge of low back pain or sciatica.

Surgical Treatment

The alternative to conservative treatment is surgery; consequently, some criteria must be established to decide when surgical intervention is indicated. The type and extent of surgery will depend on the experience, ability, and judgment of the consulting surgeon. Discussion, however, of surgical techniques is beyond the scope of this text.

Indications for Surgical Intervention. The criteria for contemplating surgical intervention can be considered as fulfilled when:

1. There is *persistent* bladder and bowel dysfunction of a neurogenic type. Rosmoff, et al, have shown that over 90 per cent of patients with lumbar nerve root compression have hypofunction of the bladder as determined by cystometry.

Insertion of a catheter to prevent overdistension of the bladder usually suffices to permit natural return of function after subsidence of the pain and radicular symptoms. If there is a persistence of bladder hypofunction after a reasonable period of conservative treatment, myelography and surgery become more imminent.

2. There is an increase in objective neurologic deficit, such as progressive weakness, increasing numbness, or increasing pain, in spite of adequate, supervised, and prolonged conservative treatment.

3. The patient is unwilling to endure the discomfort or to submit to further conservative treatment, owing to lowering of the pain-threshold, psychologic decompensation, financial reasons, or pressures beyond the control of the doctor may prompt surgical consultation. When, however, there is no bladder or bowel involvement and no progression of neurologic deficit, great care must be exercised in allowing the patient to press for surgery.

116

Surgery must be considered a *last resort* procedure in which a disk that is considered damaged beyond natural repair is removed because in this way the degeneration is surgically completed. Surgery can give no greater guarantee of relief from pain than that promised by further conservative treatment. Surgery offers no positive assurance that impaired strength to any significant degree will return; and lastly, there is no guarantee that recurrence of the condition is not again possible. Surgery frequently results in ameliorating the symptoms, but its limitation should be made known to the impatient patient who is pressing for surgery against conservative advice and may be expecting immediate results which are not predictable.

With surgical intervention *not all patients with sciatica are found to have a prolapsed disk,* and removal of a disk herniation when one is found "bulging" may give only temporary relief of symptoms. It has been estimated (Hirsch) that only 15 per cent of patients get *complete* and *permanent* relief of their pain after surgical resection of the disk herniation and nucleus.

Diskectomy followed by fusion has been advocated to ensure better and more permanent results because of the long time required for "natural" fibrous fusion after mere diskectomy. Also fusion is advocated because removal of the herniated degenerated disk leaves an unstable degenerated disk annulus.

Fusion, proven to be solid, does not guarantee permanent relief of symptoms. Patients after a "solid" fusion frequently continue to have symptoms similar to those present before surgery. X-rays cannot confirm the solidity of a fusion and only re-exploration can do so. To find a solid fusion with persistent symptomatology leaves a perplexing situation.

Fusion does not eliminate disk function nor eliminate stresses imposed upon the disk. Fusion of one space may actually place added burden upon adjacent disks, and although they were initially not the culprits they now become so. Morbidity and prolonged convalescence are greater after surgical fusion which makes it a less common practice. Convalescence is estimated between 6 to 24 months.

Selection of surgical patients, especially for fusion, must be meticulous. An unintelligent or severely psychoneurotic patient is a poor candidate. A patient more interested in litigation than in recovery is also a poor risk. Relief of the patient's symptoms from wearing an antigravity body plaster jacket (cast) for a period of four to six weeks is a good criteria that surgical fusion may be beneficial.

SUMMARY

Disk disease constitutes a specific disease entity that can be analyzed on a purely mechanical basis. The disk normally acting as a compressible weight-bearing hydraulic system permits pain and disability when its elastic properties are lost.

Narrowing of the intervertebral space because of disk degeneration causes a form of degenerative arthritis termed "spondylosis." Spondylosis is capable of causing localized low back pain, or it may irritate the emerging spinal nerve root and cause sciatica.

Herniation of a lumbar disk from its annular confinement creates a clinical syndrome the mechanics of which are clearly understandable. The level of disk herniation and the extent of herniation can be objectively determined by systematic examination.

Conservative treatment is based on correcting the mechanics that initiated the symptoms.

CHAPTER 6

Miscellaneous Low Back Conditions and Their Relationship to Low Back Discomfort and Disability

Numerous conditions of the lumbosacral spine are frequently mentioned as causes of low back discomfort and disability. A complete dissertation on these conditions is not within the scope of this text, but no treatise on low back pain would be complete without at least a mention of those most common. These conditions must be considered in the differential diagnosis when they are found to be present, and the symptoms of the patient must be attributed in some part to their presence.

SPONDYLOLISTHESIS

Spondylolisthesis is a condition of forward subluxation of the body of one vertebra on the vertebra below it. The term is derived from the Greek word *olisthesis* which means a slipping or falling. The condition of spondylolisthesis is not limited to any specific segment of the vertebral column but most commonly refers to the displacement of the last lumbar vertebra over the body of the sacrum. It is to spondylolisthesis in this location that the following discussion refers.

Since the fifth vertebra reposes on the inclined plane, it will tend to glide down the incline because of gravitational forces. Sliding is prevented in part by the angulation and the overriding of the inferior facet on the superior facet in the posterior segment of the functional unit. Other factors that maintain this relationship and prevent sliding are the adequacy of the longitudinal ligaments and the integrity of the disk to maintain sufficient intradiskal pressure to keep the longitudinal ligaments taut and the posterior articulations in their proper relationship to each other.

Spondylolisthesis most commonly occurs as a sequela to a pathologic condition of spondylolysis. The terms "spondylolisthesis" and "spondylolysis" are used together so frequently that the conditions are considered interdependent. Such a relationship is not immutable as either condition can be present in the absence of the other. Spondylolysis is a bony defect of the neural arch (Fig. 61), causing the posterior portion of the functional unit to split into two segments so that there is no longer continuity of the superior and the inferior articular

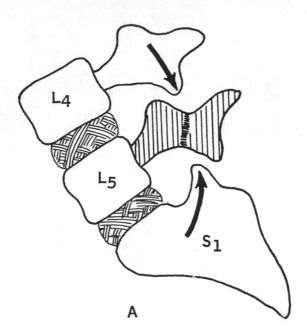

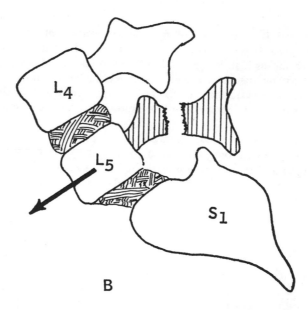

FIGURE 61. Mechanism of spondylolysis (postulated). The "pincer" effect of the adjacent facets on the interposed isthmus is demonstrated (A) with ultimate spondylolisthesis (B) due to the restraining mechanism of the posterior articulation now being detached.

processes. Part of the mechanism that normally prevents sliding is defective, and there exists the possibility of the vertebral body and its attached portion of the posterior segment pulling away from the detached fragment. The two posterior segments in spondylolysis are kept together by fibrous tissue rather than by normal bony contiguity.

The mere presence of spondylolysis does not produce any symptoms nor does it impose any functional impairment. Spondylolysis is an anatomic variant established by x-ray studies. Regarding the etiology of spondylolysis, the congenital basis, which is the most widely held theory, is not tenable since no evidence of spondylolysis with spondylolisthesis has ever been found in a fetus or in the newborn. A very low incidence of spondylolysis-spondylolisthesis is found in the age group under 10 years.

Fracture of the pars interarticularis appears as a more plausible cause. This concept envisions a fracture occurring as the result of a pincer effect of adjacent facets; for example, the inferior facet of the cephalad vertebra approaches the superior facet of the caudal vertebra and the interposed neural arch undergoes a compression fracture (Fig. 61).

Spondylolisthesis resulting from spondylolysis is not found to be greater in those between the ages of 20 to 70 years; in fact, any progression of displacement after the age of 20 is considered to be the exception. Statistically, 70 per cent of spondylolisthesis resulting from spondylolysis occurs at the fifth vertebra, 25 per cent at the fourth lumbar vertebra, and only 4 per cent at a higher level. In a reported series, only 6 per cent of patients with spondylolysis did not also have spondylolisthesis. Evidently the greatest factor in the causation of spondylolisthesis is spondylolysis of the neural arch.

Pain in the low back occurs frequently in spondylolisthesis (70 per cent), whereas sciatica is infrequent. Of a large group of patients having spondylolisthesis, studies revealed that only 10 per cent had subjective sciatica or a positive reaction to the straight leg raising test. Pain in the low back attributable to spondylolisthesis undoubtedly results from the strain imposed on the ligaments and the intervertebral joints. The presence of nerve root irritation, when it does occur, probably results from disruption of the integrity of the aperture of the intervertebral foramen. The instability of the lytic vertebra, the mechanical distortion of the foramen due to the displacement of the vertebra, and the traction on the nerve roots by the migrating vertebra may all contribute to the development of sciatica. The concept that the fibrous tissue which replaces the defect in the pars interarticularis causes compression of the nerve roots at the foramen is not substantiated by surgical exploration.

Conservative treatment for symptomatic spondylolisthesis consists of instituting methods to produce a flattened lumbar spine curve. By reduction of lumbar lordosis there is a decrease in the sacral angulation and thus the inclination of the plane upon which the lumbar vertebra rests is decreased. Decrease in the incline lessens the gravitational force which promotes slipping and thus diminishes the posterior articular approximation with its resultant synovial irritation and ligamentous strain.

In the conservative treatment, exercises to accomplish pelvic tilting are of paramount importance. Frequently a brace or a corset is required to accomplish

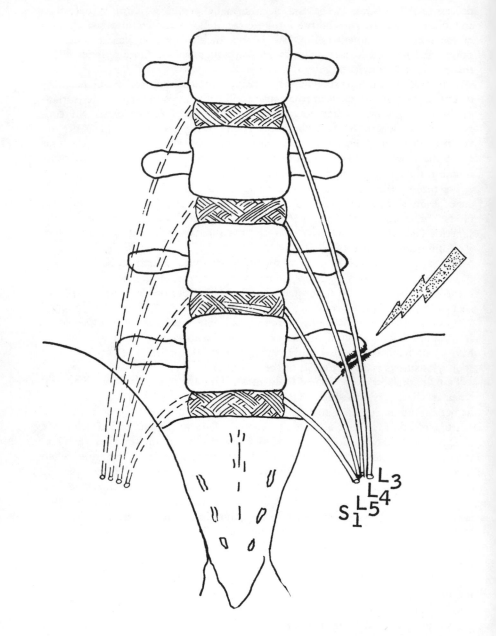

FIGURE 62. Sacralization of transverse process. The elongated left transverse process of the fifth lumbar vertebra forms a pseudoarthrosis at its point of contact with the sacral wing. The passage over the area of pseudoarthrosis of the L₃-L₄ nerve roots irritates the contiguous branches. The mechanism of pain due to mechanical irritation on left lateral flexion can be visualized.

the necessary decrease in lordosis. Such support should be worn long enough to permit healing of the posterior articular inflammation and allow enough training time in the concept of "flat back." Here again, too long a period of bracing results in ligamentous laxity as well as disuse weakness and atrophy of the musculature and in the end will defeat the purpose of the brace.

Spondylolisthesis occurring as a sequela to disk degeneration, if clinically symptomatic, has the same mechanism as does discogenic disease or spondylolysis, and the treatment obviously follows the same procedure as directed for the fore-going conditions and for similar reasons.

SACRALIZED TRANSVERSE PROCESS

Sacralization of a transverse process, a congenitally long transverse process forming a pseudo-arthrosis at its point of contact with the sacrum or the ilium, is capable of causing low back pain and sciatica. The usual level of the elongated transverse process is the fifth lumbar vertebra, and the pseudo-arthrosis is found at its tip and at the point in contact with the ipsilateral ilium.

Pain resulting from movement at the pseudoarthrosis will be caused by or be aggravated mostly during the movement of lateral flexion of the trunk, as contrasted with discogenic disease in which pain occurs during anterior-posterior movement.

Sciatic pain when it occurs because of this condition localizes at a level of the L_4 root or a higher root in the area in which the nerve root is irritated (Fig. 62). Pain is more sharply localized at the site of sacralization. Motor, sensory, and reflex changes are rare even in the presence of subjective sciatica.

The large transverse process and its sacral pseudoarthrosis must be visualized on x-ray film even to consider the feasibility of this diagnosis. The possible occurrence of a herniated lumbar disk with radiculitis in a patient whose x-rays reveal a large transverse process and a suggested pseudoarthrosis must be kept in mind.

INTRASPINAL LESION CAUSING SCIATICA

Intraspinal tumors can mimic the history and objective findings of a herniated lumbar disk. This possibility must never be overlooked. The numerous types of intraspinous lesions are frequently listed in medical literature and will not be repeated here. The true nature of a lesion, other than a herniated lumbar disk, cannot be accurately determined from the history or from the neurologic or orthopedic examination alone. Standard routine roentgenograms are not conclusive, nor usually are they even suggestive of such a diagnosis. Only by Pantopaque studies preceded by spinal fluid studies is this type of lesion suggested as a possibility.

The existence of an intraspinal lesion, other than a herniated lumbar disk, should be suspected when (1) there is a failure to respond to conservative treatment and the pain remains intractible or when there is unusual progression of the neurologic signs. This failure to respond even in probable disk trouble should lead to consideration of myelography which may then reveal the tumor. It should also be suspected when (2) neurogenic type of bladder or bowel dysfunction exists, or (3) when nocturnal pain awakens the patient and when such pain is essentially unrelated to movement, position, or activity, or (4) when the presence of upper motor neuron is involved neurologically. The presence of spasticity, hyperactive reflexes, conus, and positive Babinski signs all indicate a lesion in the central nervous system and not of the lower neuron type of involvement found in herniated disk disease. Findings not related to a single nerve root level (myotome or dermatome) should also raise doubt regarding a disk as the reason for the symptoms or the findings.

The suspicion of possible cord tumor rather than disk herniation can be confirmed by lumbar puncture, spinal fluid studies, cystometric confirmation tests of bladder function, Pantopaque myelography, and ultimately surgical exploration.

EXTRASPINAL LESIONS MIMICKING HERNIATED LUMBAR DISK

Pressure on the sciatic nerve beyond the limits of the vertebral column or distal to the intervertebral foramen must also always be considered in the differential diagnosis of nerve root impairment. Pressure on the sciatic nerve from osteoid osteoma, glomus tumors of the leg, and subfascial fat herniations can cause low back pain with the addition of subjective sciatica, and even bring about evidence of nerve root impingement. The diagnosis of these conditions may be confirmed by x-ray studies, palpation of suspicious masses, and ultimate confirmation by surgical exploration and excision.

A syndrome frequently mentioned yet rarely encountered and one that is difficult to verify accurately is the so-called "pyriformis syndrome." This syndrome is an alleged entrapment of the sciatic nerve as it passes in front of the pyriformis muscle and behind the gemelli and obturator muscles where the sciatic nerve emerges from the pelvis. The region of the entrapment is located at the exterior portion of the sciatic notch of the pelvis.

As the pyriformis muscle is an external rotator of the femur, the diagnostic feature of this syndrome should be the reproduction of sciatic pain upon straight leg raising which causes the lower extremity to be internally rotated, but there is relief upon externally rotating the leg while it is still in the SLR position. The explanation of the mechanism is that with internal rotation the pyriformis is taut and entraps the nerve in its passage. External rotation, done passively by the examiner to relax pyriformis muscle contraction, relieves the traction on the nerve.

In the differential diagnosis of the pyriformis syndrome, the gluteal muscles escape atrophy whereas lumbar radicular pressure from a disk herniation involves the gluteal muscles with resultant weakness and atrophy.

MALINGERING

The unpleasant use of the term *malingering* cannot be avoided in a discussion of low back pain with or without subjective sciatica. If malingering is alleged, the statement must imply symptoms falsified intentionally and with the deliberate purpose of attaining a gain; the symptoms are based on no organic pathology. In essence, malingering is more an accusation than a diagnosis. The decision that the symptoms are mimicked and the signs point to malingering requires, however, careful, astute evaluation.

The true malingerer is uncommon. Malingering must never be confused with anxiety, conversion hysteria, or nervousness. The symptoms that ultimately prove to be a somatization of psychic factors must be unearthed and correctly brought to the attention of the patient with the intent of helping rather than accusing. The malingerer needs to be similarly treated; then the motive must be established. Treatment of malingering understandably differs from that of emotionally induced symptoms. In the latter case too much harm could accrue from a misjudgment which may negate any benefit ultimately expected in the combined mechanical and psychologic therapy.

No laboratory tests differentiate hysterical manifestations from malingering. Only the experience of the examiner and his ability to evaluate adequately the history and the physical findings can label the malingerer. The hysteric's mimicry of symptoms may be equal to those of the malingerer and his story also equal in absurdity, but astute observers will be able to unearth the true motive.

Knowledge of normal stance and proper kinetics, an appreciation of the deviations from the normal, significant understanding of possible mechanisms capable of causing the symptoms, and most of all the realization that the patient is a human being with motivation transcending all these concepts related to the physical only will aid the doctor in arriving at a reasonable conclusion.

125

Bibliography

Armstrong, J. R.: Lumbar Disc Lesions. Pathogenesis and Treatment of Low Back Pain and Sciatica. The Williams & Wilkins Co., Baltimore, 1952.

Bailey, W.: Observations on the etiology and frequency of spondylolisthesis and its precursors. Radiol. 48: 107, 1947.

Barr, J. S.: Low back and sciatic pain. Results of treatment. J. Bone & Joint Surg. 33A: 633, 1951.

Bartelink, D. L.: The role of abdominal pressure in relieving the pressure on the lumbar intervertebral discs. J. Bone & Joint Surg. 39B: ·718, 1957.

Bradford, K. K., and Sperling, R. G.: The Intervertebral Disc, ed. 2. Charles C Thomas, Publisher, Springfield, Illinois, 1945.

Breig, A.: Biomechanics of the Central Nervous System. Year Book Medical Publishers, Chicago, 1960.

Charnley, J.; Orthopedic signs in the diagnosis of disc protrusions. Lancet 1: 186, 1951.

Colonna, P. C., and Friedenberg, Z. B.: The disc syndrome. Results of the conservative care of patients with positive myelograms. J. Bone & Joint Surg., 31A: 614, 1949.

Craig, W. McK., Svien, H. J., Dodge, H. W., and Camp, J. D.: Intraspinal lesions masquerading as protruded lumbar intervertebral disks. J.A.M.A. 149: 250, 1952.

Crisp, E. J.: In Massage, manipulation and traction. Physical Medicine Library, Vol. 5, edited by S. Licht. Elizabeth Licht, Publisher, New Haven, p. 147.

Cyriax, J. H.: Lumbago-mechanism of dural pain. Lancet 2: 427, 1955.

Dandy, W. E.: Loose cartilage from intervertebral disc simulating tumour of the spinal cord. Arch. Surg. 19: 660, 1929.

Davis, P. R.: Posture of the trunk during lifting of weights. Brit. Med. J. 1: 87, 1959.

Edgar, M. A., and Nundy, S.: Innervation of the spinal dura mater. J. Neurol. Neurosurg. & Psychiat. 29:530, 1966.

Eie, N., and Wehn, P: Measurements of the intra-abdominal pressure in relation to weight bearing of the lumbosacral spine. J. of the Oslo City Hospitals 12: 205, 1962.

Falconer, M. A., McGeorge, M., and Begg, A. C.: Observations on the cause and mechanism of symptom-production in sciatica and low back pain. J. Neurol. Neurosurg. and Psychiat. II:13, 1948.

Foerster, O.: The dermatome in man. Brain 56:1, 1933.

Friberg, S.: Studies on spondylolisthesis. Acta Chir. Scandinav. 82: (Supp 55) 1, 1939.

Friberg, S., and Hirsch, C.: Anatomical and clinical studies on lumbar disc degeneration. Acta Orthop. Scandinav. 19: 222, 1949.

Friberg, S., and Hult, L.: Comparative study of abrodil myelogram and operative findings in low back pain and sciatica. Acta. Orthop. Scandinav. 20: 303, 1951.

Goddard, M. D., and Reid, J. D.: Movements inducted by straight leg raising in the lumbosacral roots, nerves and plexus, and in the intrapelvic section of the sciatic nerve. J. Neurol. Neurosurg. & Psychiat. 28: 12, 1965.

Haas, S. L.: Fusion of vertebrae following resection of intervertebral disc. J. Bone & Joint Surg. 28: 544, 1946.

Hanraets, P.R.M.J.: The Degenerative Back. Amsterdam-New York. Elsevier Pub., 1959.

Harris, R. I., and MacNab, I.: Structural changes on lumbar intervertebral discs: Their relationship to low back pain and sciatica. J. Bone & Joint Surg. 36B:304, 1954.

Hause, F. B., and O'Connor, S. J.: Specific management for lumbar and sacral radiculitis. J.A.M.A. 166: 1285, 1958.

Haymaker, W., and Woodhall, B.: Peripheral Nerve Injuries, ed. 2. W. B. Saunders Co., Philadelphia, 1959.

Henderson, R. S.: The treatment of lumbar intervertebral disk protrusion. An assessment of conservative measures. British Med. J. 2: 597, 1952.

Hilel, N.: Spondylolysis. J. Bone & Joint Surg. 41A: 303, 1959.

Hirsch, C.: Studies on the mechanism of low back pain. Acta Orthop. Scandinav. XX: 261, 1951.

Hirsch, C.: Efficiency of surgery in low back disorders. J. Bone & Joint Surg. 47A:991, 1965.

Hirsch, C., Ingelmark, B. E., and Miller, M.: The anatomical bases for low back pain. Studies on the presence of sensory nerve endings in ligamentous, capsular and intervertebral disc structures in the human lumbar spine. Acta Orthop. Scandinav. 33: 1, 1963.

Hirsch, C.: An attempt to diagnose the level of a disc lesion clinically by disc puncture. Acta Orthop. Scandinav. 18: 132, 1948.

Hirsch, C., and Nachemson, A.: New observations on the mechanical behavior of lumbar discs. Acta Orthop. Scandinav. 23: 254, 1959.

Hirsch, C., and Schajowicz, F.: Studies on structural changes in the lumbar annulus fibrosus. Acta Orthop. Scandinav. 22: 184, 1953.

Hovelaque, A.: Le nerf sinu-vertebral. Ann. Anat. Pathol 2: 435, 1925.

Howarth, M. B., and Petrie, J. G.: Injuries of the Spine. The Williams & Wilkins Co., Baltimore, 1964.

Inman, V. T., and Saunders, J. B. de C.: The clinico-anatomical aspects of the lumbosacral region. Radiology, 38: 669, 1942.

Inman, V. T., and Saunders, J. B. de C.: Anatomical and physiological aspects of injuries of the intervertebral disc. J. Bone & Joint Surg. 29A: 461, 1947.

Jonck, L. M.: The influence of weight bearing on the lumbar spine: A radiological study. So. Africa J. Radiol. 2:25, 1964.

Kaplan, E. B.: Recurrent meningeal branch of the spinal nerves. Bull. Hosp. Joint Dis. 8:108, 1947.

Keegan, J.: Alterations of the lumbar curve related to posture and seating. J. Bone & Joint Surg. 35A: 589, 1953.

Key, J. A.: Intervertebral disk lesions are most common cause of low back pain with or without sciatica. Ann. Surg. 121: 534, 1945.

Key, J. A.: Indications for operations in disc lesions on the lumbosacral spine. Ann. Surg. 135: 886, 1952.

Keyes, D. C., and Compere, E. L.: The normal and pathological physiology of the nucleus pulposus of the intervertebral disc. J. Bone & Joint Surg. 14:897, 1932.

Knutsson, B.: Electromyographic studies in the diagnosis of lumbar disc herniations. Acta Orthop. Scandinav. 28: 290, 1959.

Knutsson, B., Lindh, K., and Telhag, H.: Sitting—An electromyographic and mechanical study. Acta Orthop. Scandinav. 37: 415, 1966.

Knutsson, F.: The instability associated with disc degeneration in the lumbar spine. Acta Radiol. Scandinav. 25: 593, 1944.

Kraft, G. L., and Leventhal, D. H.: Facet synovial impingement: A new concept in the etiology of lumbar vertebral derangement. Surg. Gynec. & Obst. 93: 439, 1951.

Laseque, C.: Considerations sur la sciatique. Archives Generales de Medicine 2: 558, 1864.

Lindahl, O.: Hyperalgesia of the lumbar nerve roots in sciatica. Acta. Orthop. Scandinav. 37:367, 1966.

Lucas, O. B.: Spinal bracing. In Orthotics Etcetera, Physical Medicine Library, Vol. 9, edited by S. Licht, Elizabeth Licht, Publisher, New Haven, 1966, p. 275.

McCrae, D. L.: Asymptomatic disk protrusions. Acta Radiologica 46: 9, 1955.

Mennell, J. McM.: Back Pain. Little Brown and Co., Boston, 1960.

Mensor, M. C.: Non-operative treatment, including manipulation for lumbar intervertebral disc syndrome. J. Bone & Joint Surg. 37A:925, 1955.

Meyerding, H. W.: The low backache and sciatic pain associated with spondylolisthesis and protruded intervertebral disc; incidence, significance, and treatment. J. Bone & Joint Surg. 23: 461, 1941.

Mixter, W. J., and Barr, J. S.: Rupture of the intervertebral disc with involvement of the spinal canal. New Eng. J. Med. 211: 210, 1934.

Morris, J. M., and Lucas, D. B.: Physiological consideration in bracing of the spine. Orthop. & Prosthetic Appliance J.: (Mar.) 1963.

Morris, J. M. and Lucas, D. B.: Biomechanics of spinal bracing. Arizona Med. 21: 170, 1964.

Morris, J. M., Lucas, D. B., and Breslar, B.: The role of the trunk in stability of the spine. J. Bone & Joint Surg. 43A: 327, 1966.

Nachemson, A.: Lumbar intradiscal pressure. Experimental studies on post-mortem material. Acta Orthop. Scandinav. Supp. 43: 1, 1960.

Nachemson, A.: The effect of forward leaning on lumbar intradiscal pressure. Acta Orthop. Scandinav. 35: 314, 1965.

Nachemson, A.: In vivo discometry in lumbar discs with irregular nucleograms. Acta Orthop. Scandinav. 36: 418, 1965.

O'Connell, J. E. A.: The indication for and results of the excision of lumbar intervertebral disc protrusions. A review of 500 cases. Ann. Roy. Coll. Surg. Eng. 6: 403, 1950.

Rabinowitch, R.: Diseases of intervertebral disc and its surrounding tissues. Charles C Thomas Publisher, Springfield, Illinois, 1961.

Reynolds, F. C., McGinnis, A. E., and Morgan, H. C.: Surgery in the treatment of low back pain and sciatica: A follow-up study. J. Bone & Joint Surg. 41A: 223, 1959.

Roofe, P. G.: Innervation of the annulus fibrosus and the posterior longitudinal ligament. Arch. Neurol. and Psychiat. 44: 100, 1940.

Rosmoff, H. L., John, J. D. H., Gallo, A. E., Ludmer, M., Givens, F. T., Carney, F. T., and Kuehn, C. A.: Cystometry in the evaluation of nerve root compression in the lumbar spine. Surg., Gynec., & Obst. 117: 263, 1963.

Smyth, J. J., and Wright, V.: Sciatica and the intervertebral disc. An experimental study. J. Bone & Joint Surg. 40A: 1401, 1958.

Soren, A.: Spondylolisthesis and allied conditions. Am. J. Orthop. 8: 8, 1966.

Spurling, R. G., and Granthan, E. G.: Ruptured discs in lower lumbar region. Am. J. Surg. 75:14, 1948.

Steindler, A.: Lectures on the Interpretation of Pain in Orthopedic Practice. Charles C Thomas, Publisher, Springfield, Illinois, 1959.

Steindler, A.: Kinesiology of the Human Body. Charles C Thomas, Publisher, Springfield, Illinois, 1955.

Taylor, T. K. F.: Treatment of lumbar disc prolapse. Am. Acad. Gen. Practice XXXII: 141, 1965.

Thieme, F. P.: Lumbar breakdown caused by erect posture on man: With emphasis on spondylolisthesis and herniated intervertebral disc. Anthropological Papers No. 4; Museum of Anthropology, 1950.

Von Luschka, H.: Die Halbgelenke des menschlichen Korpers. Vol. 4. G. Reimer, Berlin, 1858.

Wiberg, G.: Back pain in relation to the nerve supply of the intervertebral disc. Acta Orthop. Scandinav. 19: 211, 1949.

Williams, P. C.: Conservative management of lesions of lumbosacral spine. In Instructional Course Lectures, edited by J. W. Edwards. American Academy of Orthop. Surgeons, Michigan, 1953, pp. 90-121:

Williams, P. C.: Examination and conservative treatment for disc lesions of lower spine. Clin. Orthop. 5: 28, 1955.

Wilson, J. C., Jr.: Degenerative arthritis of lumbar intervertebral joints, a clinical study. Am. J. Surg. 100:313, 1960.

Wilson, J. C.: Low back pain and sciatica. J.A.M.A. 200: 705, 1967.

Woolsey, R. D.: Mechanism of neurological symptoms and signs in spondylolisthesis at fifth lumbar, first sacral level. J. Neurosurg. 11:67, 1954.

Wright, J.: Mechanics in relation to derangement of the facet joints of the spine. Arch. Phys. Therap. 25: 201, 1944.

Index

Lumbar region
  disk herniation in, 85-118
  facets of, 8
  lordosis of, 10, 13, 33
  spasm of, flattening with, 97
Lumbosacral angle, 20, 33-40
Luschka, recurrent nerve of, 87

MALINGERING, 102, 125
Medicolegal aspects, 91, 107
Meningeal nerve, recurrent, 87
Muscle spasm, 19
  relaxation of, 110
Muscular support of spine, 26-30
Myelography, 107, 124
Myotome testing, 103

NECK. See Cervical spine.
Nerve, pressure on, 92
Nerve root irritation, 39, 84, 92
Nerves, sensory, 18
Neurogenic bladder, 116, 124
Newborn, spine of, 14
Nucleus pulposus, 2, 4
Numbness in disk herniation, 91, 92

OSTEOARTHRITIS, 107
Osteoma, osteoid, 124
Osteophyte formation, 107

PAIN
  in lumbar disk herniation, 85-86
  in tissues, sites of, 17, 18-19
  ligamentous stretch, 45
  localization of, 49-57
  nocturnal, 124
  referred, 89
Pantopaque study, 107, 123, 124
Pelvic angle, 28
Pelvis, 10
  lumbar-pelvic rhythm, 23-26, 31, 44,
    53-56, 71-73
  obliquity of, 30, 52, 74
  rotation of, 12, 23-26
  tilting of, 12, 13
    exercises for, 59-61
  traction of, 112-113
  tucked in, 58, 74
Position in bed rest, 109
Posterior longitudinal ligament, 17, 18
Posture, 1, 10, 14-18
  chair-sitting, 72-73
  emotional tone affecting, 16, 50, 59, 82
  evaluation of, 51
  faulty, correction of, 58-59

flat back, 71
  standing, 72
Pregnancy, low back pain in, 39
Pseudoarthrosis, 39, 123
Psoas muscle, 61
Pyriformis syndrome, 124

QUADRICEPS muscle, testing of, 105

RADICULITIS, sciatic, 92
Radiologic studies, 106-107, 123
Reflexes, testing of, 105
Roentgenography, 106-107, 123
Rotation of pelvis, 12, 23-26
Rupture. See Herniation.

SACRAL angle, 12-13, 37
Sacralized transverse process, 122-123
Sacroiliac region, dimples in, 52
Sacrum, 10
Sciatic nerve
  entrapment of, 124
  pressure on, from extraspinal lesions,
    124
  root of, 19
Sciatica, 65, 84, 85, 86, 87
  crossed response and, 102
Sclerosis, marginal, 107
Scoliosis, 42
  acute protective, 99
  functional, 31, 44, 54, 77
  in lumbar disk herniation, 90, 95
  structural, 31, 42, 77
Sedatives, use of, 110
Sensory examination, 106
Shearing stress, 33, 80
Side-bending, 28
Sinu vertebralis nerve, 87
Sneezing, leg pain with, 95
Spasm
  iliopsoas, 85
  lumbar, 97
  muscular, 19
    relaxation of, 110
Spinal fluid studies, 124
Spinal fusion, 117
Spine, 1-10
  cervical. See Cervical spine.
  extension of, 20-23
    two-stage, 44
  kinetic. See Kinetic spine.
  kissing, 39
  pain-sensitive tissues of, 17, 18-19
  static. See Static spine.
Spondylolisthesis, 119-123

133

Spondylolysis, 108, 119
Spondylosis, 82
Spur, arthritic, 82, 84, 107
Standing posture, 72
Static spine, 1, 8, 10-18
    examination of, 51-53
    pain in, 33-40
Strain, ligamentous, 26
Stress
    abnormal, on normal back, 42
    normal
        on abnormal back, 42-46
        on unprepared normal back, 46-48
    shearing, 33, 80
Stretch pain, ligamentous, 45
Stretching exercises. *See* Exercises.
Surgery in lumbar disk herniation,
    116-117
Sway back, 33, 38, 56
Synovial tissues
    and fluid, 8, 19
    inflammation of, 38
Synovitis, articular, acute and chronic,
    82-84, 92

TEARS in annulus, 90
Tendon reflexes, 106
Tension, effects on disks, 80-82
Tensor fascia lata, 28, 77
Test(s)
    ankle flexion, 101

confirmatory, in disk disease, 106-107
    neurologic, 103-106
    sensory, 106
    straight leg raising, 100
Thoracic curve, 10
Thoracic facets, 8
Tibialis anterior muscle testing, 103
Tight low back mechanism, 45
Tightness of hamstrings, 44, 53, 54
Tilting of pelvis, 12, 13
    exercise for, 59-61
Traction, 111-113
Tranquilizing drugs, 110
Transverse process, sacralization of, 123
Treatment
    for correction of faulty mechanics,
        58-77
    of herniated lumbar disk, 108-113
Tumors
    extradural, of spine, 108
    glomus, of leg, 124
    intraspinal, 123
Two-stage extension of spine, 44

VASCULAR supply to disk, 5
Vertebral bodies, anatomy of, 2

X-RAY studies, 106-107, 123, 124

"Y" LIGAMENT, 26
Yoga position, 64